Alive **Natural Health Guides**

Superfoods

NATURE'S TOP TEN

Myrna Chandler Goldstein, MA
Mark Allan Goldstein, MD

books
Alive

Summertown
TENNESSEE

CONTENTS

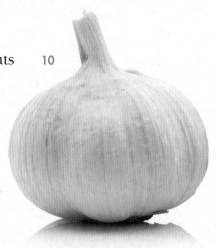

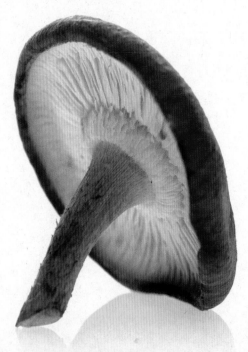

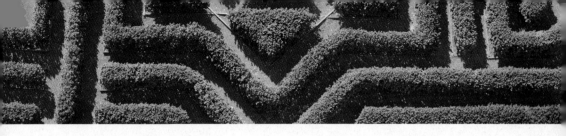

INTRODUCTION

It has long been acknowledged that the quality of health we enjoy is largely dependent upon the foods we eat. The foods described in this book are superheroes that can usher us all to safety by preventing—and even reversing—chronic diseases, bolstering our immune systems, and contributing to long life. Of all the foods that are protective, berries, broccoli and broccoli sprouts, cranberries, flaxseeds, garlic, kale, mushrooms, onions, sea vegetables, soybeans, and turmeric stand out from the crowd as having the most solid scientific research proving their definitive health benefits. Unless you have an intolerance or allergy to these foods, we encourage you to consume them as often as possible.

Nutrition information can be conflicting and confusing. However, there's little controversy when the discussion centers around fresh whole foods like those described in this book. Blueberries, for instance, appear on every superfoods list we know of. If you choose your information (like your food) carefully, you can greatly improve your odds for enjoying a long, healthy life.

Many people have empowered themselves by making healthful food choices, and we're no different. We've changed our diets considerably over time as we learned more. We had a long way to go: Like so many in our generation, we didn't give a second thought to nutrition when we were younger. Rather, we tended to stick with the familiar foods that our families traditionally ate. We thought it was important to have meat on the table and to consume large amounts of milk and eggs, as was recommended at the time. It turns out that this "affluent" diet was actually more costly, at least in terms of health, than we ever dreamed, but scientists were beginning to make the connection.

We couldn't do much about the fact that we both had a parent or sibling who had colorectal cancer, but we knew we had to improve our diets to avoid the same fate. Members on both sides of our family also had elevated levels of cholesterol and high blood pressure, dangerous contributors to cardiovascular disease. Today, cancer and cardiovascular disease are the leading causes of death in the United States. Both are chronic diseases that have affected virtually every family we know.

Wouldn't it be wonderful if we could protect our loved ones from experiencing these diseases?

While working on numerous books and articles about food and nutrition, we repeatedly uncovered evidence that certain foods are packed with vital nutrients that protect us from illness. The superfoods we recommend are all plant-based foods, and most are extremely low in fat. They're also rich in antioxidants, carbohydrates, minerals, and vitamins. Antioxidants are substances that help neutralize free radicals, which are unstable molecules that have been linked to chronic illnesses, such as cancer, heart disease, and Alzheimer's disease. In addition, these superfoods are packed with fiber, which helps protect us from disease in many ways. For example, fiber is essential for removing cancer-causing toxins from the gastrointestinal tract, and it also rids the body of excess cholesterol.

In the recipe section of this book, you'll see examples of how our favorite superfoods can be prepared. We hope these ideas help you get started, but feel free to experiment and find new and different ways to include superfoods in your everyday meals. All of the recipe ingredients are readily available and can become staples in your kitchen.

Now's the time to begin. Let superfoods lead the way to superhealth!

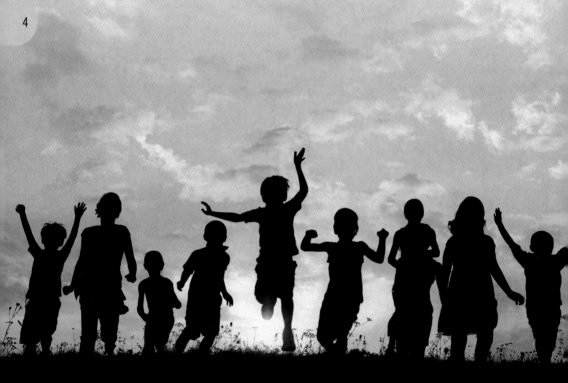

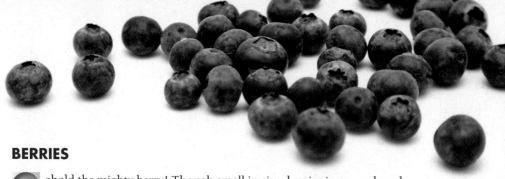

BERRIES

Behold the mighty berry! Though small in size, berries in general, and blueberries and cranberries in particular, are powerfully nutritious superfoods that contain great amounts of antioxidants. These health-boosting phytochemicals protect against cancer, cardiovascular disease, and many other ailments. The ripest berries have the most antioxidants.

Both blueberries and cranberries are native to North America, and Native Americans are credited with introducing these healthful fruits to early settlers. In addition to eating the berries, Native Americans relied on them for their medicinal properties. One common practice, for example, was to apply cranberries to arrow wounds. Today we know that cranberries have antimicrobial and anti-inflammatory properties.

About 90 percent of the world's blueberries are grown in the United States and Canada, and these tiny fruits have tremendous bragging rights. For example, just one-half cup of blueberries—about seventy-five wild blueberries or forty to forty-five cultivated blueberries—has 7 milligrams of vitamin C, which helps the body use protein, heal wounds, and absorb iron. Vitamin C is also important for a healthy immune system. Since the body is unable to store vitamin C, daily intake is essential. Furthermore, blueberries are an excellent source of manganese, which is needed for bone development and for converting the proteins, carbohydrates, and fats in foods into energy. And last but not least, one-half cup of blueberries has 1.8 grams of dietary fiber. Most people don't get enough fiber in their diets, which is unfortunate because a higher intake of fiber improves digestion, decreases cholesterol levels, and protects against heart disease and type 2 diabetes.

One reason that cranberries are superfoods is because they have more antioxidants than other common fruits. In fact, cranberries have been found to have the highest total content of phenols (a type of antioxidant). Cranberries also contain vitamins C, K, and E, as well as fiber and manganese. Generations of people have used cranberries to prevent and treat urinary tract infections. Moreover, cranberries support cardiovascular health and have anticancer and anti-inflammatory properties.

Like many other superfoods, berries are loaded with nutrients but are extremely low in calories and fat. One-half cup of blueberries has only 41 calories and the same amount of cranberries, with only 30 calories, has

HOW TO FREEZE FRESH BERRIES

Arrange washed fresh berries in a single layer on a baking sheet and put the baking sheet in the freezer. After a few hours, when the berries are frozen, remove the baking sheet from the freezer and transfer the berries to ziploc bags or plastic containers before returning them to the freezer, where they will keep for up to one year.

even fewer. And all berries have essentially no fat and can be enjoyed in many ways. Fresh, frozen, or dried berries can be added to smoothies or baked goods. Most berries are delicious fresh, just as they are, or added to salads or cereals. Cranberries, however, are too tart to be comfortably consumed fresh and whole, so they're often used in the manufacture of juice cocktails or sauces. Many of these commercial products contain excessive amounts of corn syrup or undesirable sweeteners. Even dried cranberries contain sugar or other sweeteners.

To avoid the sweeteners typically added to cranberry products, purchase 100 percent fruit juices (cranberries may be blended with other, sweeter fruits in these natural juices) or buy fresh cranberries and incorporate them into dishes made with other whole foods. For example, fresh or frozen cranberries can be used in blended juices or smoothies, with dates or other fruits added for sweetener. In the fall, fresh cranberries are available in most supermarket produce sections and can be frozen for up to one year (see sidebar, above).

Cranberries grow on vines in impermeable beds that are layered with sand, peat, gravel, and clay. These beds are known as bogs. One harvest method is to flood the beds and collect the berries from the water; people who have seen this process may assume cranberries are grown in water, but that's not the case. The fruits that are harvested by water are typically used to make juice and processed foods. Cranberries that are sold fresh in the supermarket produce section are typically picked by hand or machine between mid-September and mid-November.

Peak times for fresh blueberries range from May to August. The blueberries are generally sold in pint or half-pint containers. One pint of fresh blueberries contains about two cups, or about four servings. Whenever possible, select organic blueberries. Conventionally grown blueberries are cultivated with large quantities of pesticides.

If you're lucky enough to have access to blueberry bushes, it's good to know that the berries reach their peak ripeness in two to three days after turning blue. Freshly picked but unwashed blueberries will keep in the refrigerator for about ten days; those purchased in a store might not

BLUEBERRIES	½ CUP
Calories	41
Fat	5%
Carbohydrates	92%
Protein	3%

CRANBERRIES	½ CUP
Calories	30
Fat	0%
Carbohydrates	100%
Protein	0%

last as long because these berries are not as fresh and have a tendency to become moldy. When blueberries are in season, try freezing them (see sidebar, previous page). When you can't get your hands on fresh blueberries, look for frozen blueberries in the grocery store.

Cancer

Many researchers have found cranberries to have anticancer properties. One researcher at the University of Massachusetts in Dartmouth reviewed the literature and found that numerous laboratory studies demonstrated the effects of cranberries against brain, breast, colon, liver, ovarian, and prostate cancer. Researchers have worked to isolate the effective chemicals in cranberries, but they acknowledge that the various healthful phytochemicals in cranberries appear to work together, meaning that the whole fruit and whole-fruit extracts, rather than isolated compounds, are most effective. The review also showed that cranberries have antimicrobial and anti-inflammatory properties.

A study based at the University of Alabama examined the ability of cranberry juice to prevent bladder cancer in rats. After chemically inducing bladder cancer in rats, the researchers found that the rats that were given cranberry juice had fewer and smaller cancerous growths.

Cardiovascular Health

Some good advice for people with cardiovascular problems, particularly those who are concerned about blocked arteries, is to eat blueberries.

Researchers at the University of Arkansas for Medical Sciences performed a study on mice raised to develop atherosclerotic lesions, which are more commonly known as plaques or fatty deposits. The mice were divided into two groups. For twenty weeks, the mice in one group were fed a diet that included fresh blueberries; the mice in the other group consumed no blueberries. At the end of the study, plaque measurements were taken at two sites on the subjects' aortas. In both locations, the plaque deposits in the mice that were given blueberries were significantly smaller: the lesions at one site were 58 percent smaller, and those at the other site were 39 percent smaller.

Memory Improvement

Blueberries are also helpful for older adults with memory problems, a concern that is increasingly more common as people live longer. Researchers based at the University of Cincinnati Academic Health Center assembled a group of nine older adults with early memory changes. For twelve weeks, the volunteers consumed wild blueberry juice every day. The group showed significant improvement on learning and memory tests, and the researchers concluded that consistent blueberry consumption could potentially ward off the neurodegeneration that leads to memory loss.

Urinary Tract Infections

A number of research studies have demonstrated cranberry juice to be effective in preventing urinary tract infections. In a study based at the University of British Columbia in Vancouver, Canada, researchers studied the effects of cranberry juice on children who had a history of urinary tract infections. To be included in the study, subjects had to be age eighteen or younger and have had at least two documented urinary tract infections during the previous year. The researchers randomly assigned forty subjects to one of two groups. Both groups were given cranberry juice daily for one year. One group received cranberry juice with high concentrations of proanthocyanidins, and the other group received cranberry juice with no proanthocyanidins. (Proanthocyanidins are the most likely compounds in cranberry juice to have antibacterial properties.) At the end of one year, the children taking the cranberry juice with proanthocyanidins had an average of 0.4 urinary tract infections; those drinking the cranberry juice without proanthocyanidins had an average of 1.15 infections. The researchers concluded that cranberry juice with high concentrations of proanthocyanidins was useful in the prevention of urinary tract infections, without fever, in children.

USING WARFARIN?

Some research has indicated that it may be dangerous for people on the blood-thinning medication warfarin to consume cranberry products. If you use warfarin, check with your medical provider before eating foods containing cranberries or drinking cranberry juice.

Numerous research studies have been designed to identify how cranberry consumption affects urinary tract infections. In several studies, results have shown that cranberry juice binds with bacteria, including E. coli. This binding action prevents microbes from attaching to cell walls, which causes infection. One study, for example, demonstrated that cranberry supplementation prevented infection from *Klebsiella pneumoniae*. In a two-phase study, researchers at the School of Medicine at the University of California, Irvine, recruited subjects who didn't have urinary tract infections and weren't taking antibiotics. During the first phase of the study, subjects collected their first urine of the day and took cranberry supplements. Over the next six hours, additional urine samples were collected every two hours. During the second phase, nine subjects collected urine samples for two days. On the second day of the phase 2 study, the subjects took cranberry supplementation. The researchers found antimicrobial activity against the bacterium *Klebsiella pneumoniae* in the urine of six of the nine subjects in phase 2.

Weight Loss

Researchers at Texas Woman's University in Denton, Texas, found that blueberries may provide a long-awaited solution for people who need to lose weight. Excess weight is a serious health concern because it puts people at increased risk for cardiovascular disease, type 2 diabetes, and some types of cancer, such as breast cancer.

In laboratory tests, the researchers applied various concentrations of wild blueberry extract to tissue cultures. They found that fat cells were more likely to break down when exposed to blueberry polyphenols (the antioxidants found in plant chemicals), and the breakdown was greater when larger concentrations of polyphenols were used. This means that on the molecular level, blueberry polyphenols appear to inhibit obesity and may also block the development of new fat cells.

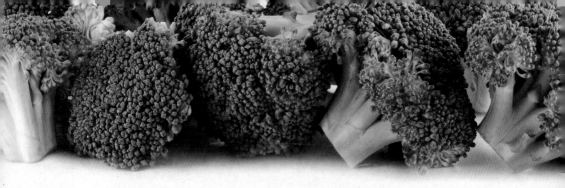

BROCCOLI AND BROCCOLI SPROUTS

For generations, children have been told to eat their broccoli, and with good reason. Broccoli has a seemingly endless list of nutrients. It's especially rich in fiber, protein, and the essential amino acid tryptophan. The vegetable also is a source of many vitamins, including A, C, E, K, folate, choline, and other B vitamins. And broccoli is no slacker when it comes to minerals; this king of vegetables is rich in calcium, iron, magnesium, manganese, molybdenum, phosphorus, potassium, and selenium.

Very few foods can compete with broccoli's royal status, except perhaps for its young relative, broccoli sprouts. One reason the sprouts are gaining so much acclaim is because they're extraordinarily rich in sulforaphane, which stimulates the production of enzymes that fight cancer. Sure, all cruciferous vegetables, including arugula, broccoli, Brussels sprouts, cabbage, cauliflower, and horseradish, are rich in sulforaphane. However, according to research done at Johns Hopkins University, in comparison with broccoli, broccoli sprouts have twenty to fifty times the amount of sulforaphane and other helpful compounds that combat cancer. In fact, eating small quantities of broccoli sprouts may be as effective in curbing cancer as consuming much larger quantities of the mature vegetable. In addition, sulforaphane protects against diabetes and microbial infection. And in general, cruciferous vegetables offer a host of other health advantages, such as lowering blood pressure and improving kidney function.

Regrettably, not everyone is a broccoli fan. For example, the first President Bush had a widely publicized disdain for this vegetable. Reportedly, his mother insisted he eat lots of broccoli when he was young. Decades later, he still had not forgotten or forgiven her, and as an adult he refused to include broccoli in his diet.

Originally cultivated in Italy, fresh broccoli is readily available throughout the year in the produce sections of US markets. Broccoli sprouts can easily be grown at home from seed (see Resources, page 62); ready-to-eat sprouts may be available in well-stocked markets and natural food stores.

	BROCCOLI, 1 CUP	BROCCOLI SPROUTS, 1 CUP
Calories	31	35
Fat	9%	14%
Carbohydrates	70%	62%
Protein	21%	24%

Both the mature vegetable and the sprout are more nutritious when eaten raw; however, if you cook them for just a few minutes, almost all their nutrients will be retained. In addition, broccoli sprouts can easily wilt when exposed to high heat. Take care not to overcook these foods, but keep in mind that large broccoli spears need more cooking time than tiny florets.

At times, fresh broccoli may be pricy. Frozen broccoli is an excellent alternative, providing it's been packaged without salt and other unnecessary ingredients. Check the label.

Cancer

Hoping to learn more about the anticancer properties of sulforaphane, researchers from the United Arab Emirates used this compound in laboratory experiments. The scientists treated human cervical cancer cells with several different concentrations of sulforaphane, both alone and in combination with gemcitabine, a chemotherapy medication used to treat some types of cancer. The researchers found that after twenty-four hours, sulforaphane induced the death of the cancer cells. Larger concentrations of sulforaphane resulted in more cell death. When they combined sulforaphane with gemcitabine, the researchers observed significant increases in cell death, and these increases were greater when larger amounts of the drug were used. The researchers concluded that, along with conventional drugs, the sulforaphane found in broccoli and broccoli sprouts is not only useful for the prevention of cancer but also for the treatment of cancer.

Researchers at Roswell Park Cancer Institute in Buffalo, New York, conducted a study on 239 people with bladder cancer. The subjects completed questionnaires on their intake of specific foods. During an average of eight years of follow-up, 179 subjects died. Of these deaths, 101 were from bladder cancer. The researchers observed that the study subjects who consumed the most broccoli, especially raw broccoli, were much more likely to survive. In their conclusion, the researchers theorized that the consumption of broccoli may improve survival from bladder cancer.

CHOOSE SPROUTS, NOT SUPPLEMENTS

Some researchers have used broccoli sprout supplements or powder with good results. If you're considering this convenient option, be aware that researchers at Oregon State University's Linus Pauling Institute have found supplements to be significantly less effective than broccoli sprouts. That's because one important enzyme, myrosinase, which is present in fresh broccoli sprouts, was missing from most of the supplements. When this enzyme is absent, the body absorbs far fewer beneficial compounds.

Cardiovascular Health

In a study conducted in Iran and at the University of Saskatchewan in Canada, researchers studied rats to determine the effect of broccoli sprouts on heart health. The rats were divided into two groups; one group ate a regular diet and the other ate a diet that included 2 percent dried broccoli sprouts. After the rats were on this diet for only ten days, their hearts were subjected to a decrease in blood supply for twenty minutes and then an increase in blood supply for two hours. The researchers examined the hearts following this procedure. In the rats that had consumed the dried broccoli sprouts, the researchers found significantly less injury to the hearts from cell death and oxidative damage. The researchers also noted that in addition to sulforaphane, broccoli sprouts have other phytochemicals that may have provided extra protection.

People with type 2 diabetes are at increased risk for cardiovascular problems, such as elevated cholesterol levels and atherosclerosis. Researchers at several locations in Iran wanted to learn if incorporating broccoli sprouts into the diet would be useful for this population, and they designed a study that enrolled 81 people with type 2 diabetes. The subjects were divided into three groups. For four weeks, the subjects in two of the groups consumed different doses of broccoli sprout powder; the subjects in the third group took placebos. Seventy-two people completed the trial. Those taking the higher dose of broccoli sprout powder experienced a number of improvements in cardiovascular health, such as decreases in serum triglycerides and increases in HDL, or "good" cholesterol. (See sidebar, above, for more information about broccoli sprout supplements.)

Chronic Obstructive Pulmonary Disease

Researchers at the National Heart and Lung Institute in London have found that eating broccoli may be useful for people with chronic obstructive pulmonary disease (COPD), an illness that makes it hard to breathe and worsens over time. Most COPD patients smoke or used to smoke; the disease encompasses both emphysema and chronic bronchitis. In one particularly challenging form of COPD, there is a decrease in lung concentrations of a protein called Nrf2, which defends the lungs against injury from inflammation. Since the sulforaphane in broccoli stabilizes Nrf2 levels in the lungs, the regular consumption of broccoli may mitigate the symptoms experienced by people with this form of COPD.

Helicobacter pylori Infection

Researchers from Johns Hopkins University in Baltimore, Maryland, and from Japan noted that the *Helicobacter pylori* infection that causes gastritis and ulcers has been strongly associated with the development of stomach cancer. To learn whether broccoli sprouts could help control this infection, they investigated the possibility in mice and infected human volunteers.

In the mouse study, the researchers found that when mice were given broccoli sprout smoothies for eight weeks, there was a fourfold increase in two of the enzymes that protect cells from oxidative damage. Moreover, the amount of stomach infection decreased by almost a hundredfold, and the amount of stomach inflammation decreased by more than 50 percent.

In the human trials, the researchers gave twenty-five people infected with *Helicobacter pylori* 2.5 ounces (70 grams) of broccoli sprouts daily for two months; another group of twenty-five infected people were given an equivalent amount of alfalfa sprouts for the same time period. The researchers checked the severity of the infections at the beginning of the trial, at four and eight weeks, and eight weeks after the trial ended. Two subjects in the alfalfa group didn't complete the trial, so the final analyses were based on the findings from forty-eight subjects.

The researchers found that the subjects who ate the broccoli sprouts experienced 40 percent reductions in their levels of HpSA, a measurement of the presence of *Helicobacter pylori* in the stools of infected people. The subjects who ate alfalfa had no change in HpSA levels. However, it's important to note that eight weeks after the subjects stopped eating broccoli sprouts, their HpSA levels returned to their pretreatment values. While broccoli sprouts failed to eradicate infections, they significantly reduced them. Therefore, the researchers concluded that the sulforaphane in broccoli sprouts is an antibacterial agent against *Helicobacter pylori*, and it can also help prevent the development of stomach cancer.

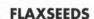

FLAXSEEDS

Flax was one of the earliest domesticated crops, and this flowering plant has long been used to produce fibers for rope and fine cloth. While the seeds have been consumed since ancient times, today we know much more about the outstanding nutrition they provide. Rich in phytochemicals, fiber, healthy fats, and protein, flaxseeds are also plentiful in minerals and vitamins. These include copper, manganese, magnesium, phosphorus, potassium, and zinc along with B vitamins, vitamin E, and folate.

Flaxseeds contain great quantities of lignans, which are phytochemicals that can provide protection from hormone-dependent cancers, such as breast and prostate cancer. Flaxseeds can also help relieve the symptoms associated with menopause.

In addition to being powerful antioxidants, lignans provide water-soluble fiber that promotes a healthy gastrointestinal tract. Many people use flaxseeds to alleviate constipation and improve regularity. However, because flaxseeds have the potential to trigger gastrointestinal symptoms, such as bloating, it's best to incorporate them into your diet slowly, gradually increasing the amount over time.

The healthy fats in flaxseeds are omega-3 fatty acids, especially alpha-linolenic acid. Omega-3 fatty acids are essential for heart health because they decrease blood pressure, inflammation, and oxidative stress. They also play crucial roles in brain function and normal growth and development. Because the body is unable to make omega-3 fatty acids, we must obtain them from food.

Flaxseeds, which can be gold or brown, are generally sold whole or ground. Whole flaxseeds are difficult to digest, so grind them before use to get the full nutritional benefits. Whole flaxseeds are protected by hard shells, so they have a much longer shelf life than ground flaxseeds, which can become rancid when the delicate oils they contain are exposed to oxygen. Therefore, you may want to purchase whole seeds and grind small amounts at a time (perhaps a one-week supply). The best way to grind flaxseeds is in a coffee grinder that's used only for flaxseeds (otherwise, the ground seeds will taste like coffee) or in a blender.

While whole flaxseeds are best stored in the freezer, a small amount of ground flaxseeds will keep for several days in a tightly sealed container in the refrigerator. The ground flaxseeds are then ready to be

FLAXSEEDS	3 TABLESPOONS
Calories	90
Fat	62%
Carbohydrates	24%
Protein	14%

added to smoothies, cereals, or salads. They can also be used in baked goods, such as breads and cookies. Although the omega-3 fatty acids in flaxseeds are sensitive to heat, the interior temperatures of most baked goods are not high enough to damage these fats.

Cancer

In a multisite trial based at the University of Texas MD Anderson Cancer Center, researchers compared the effects of a flaxseed-rich diet and a low-fat diet in men diagnosed with prostate cancer. The researchers recruited 161 subjects who were candidates for prostate gland removal and divided the men into four groups. The men in the control group ate their usual diets, the men in the second group ate a diet supplemented with flaxseeds, the men in the third group ate a low-fat diet, and the men in the fourth group ate a low-fat diet supplemented with flaxseeds. On average, the subjects remained on the diets for thirty days. The researchers found that the men taking supplemental flaxseeds had slower-growing prostate cancer.

German researchers evaluated the ability of dietary lignans, such as flaxseed lignans, to protect against cancer. Flaxseed lignans are metabolized into enterolignans, so the researchers studied the enterolignan levels in a group of 1,140 postmenopausal women between the ages of fifty and seventy-four who were diagnosed with breast cancer. They found that the women with the highest levels of enterolactone (a biomarker for dietary lignans) had a significantly lower risk for death. In fact, their mortality rates were reduced by two-fifths compared to the women with the lowest levels of enterolactone. Moreover, high levels of enterolactone offered protection against the spread of cancer and the formation of secondary tumors.

Cardiovascular Health

In a study conducted at the James R. Randall Research Center at the Archer Daniels Midland Company in Decatur, Illinois, and in China, researchers tested the ability of flaxseeds to lower cholesterol and glucose (sugar) levels in subjects with elevated cholesterol levels. Sixty-six subjects were randomly assigned to take supplemental flaxseed lignan extract or a placebo. At the end of eight weeks, fifty-five subjects completed the trial. The researchers found that the subjects taking the flaxseed lignan extract experienced significant reductions in total cholesterol and LDL, or "bad" cholesterol, levels. After fasting for at least eight hours, the subjects also had lower concentrations of glucose in the blood.

A trial at the University of Copenhagen in Denmark tested the theory that adding flaxseed fiber to the diet would lower blood cholesterol and also increase fat excretion. Ten women and seven men were recruited and assigned to three groups. Each group was fed a different diet: one that included a flaxseed drink, one that included flaxseed-fiber bread, and one that was low in fiber. All the food was supplied by the researchers. Compared to the low-fiber diet, the flaxseed-drink diet lowered total cholesterol and LDL by 12 percent and 15 percent, respectively. The flaxseed-bread diet lowered total cholesterol and LDL by 7 percent and 9 percent respectively. Both diets produced increases in fecal fat excretion (fat in the stool).

To conduct their tests on flaxseeds, researchers in Japan recruited thirty men between the ages of twenty-one and fifty-seven. All of the subjects had slightly elevated cholesterol levels. During a twelve-week study, the subjects were randomly divided into three treatment groups. The subjects in two of the groups received different doses of flaxseed lignan extract daily; the subjects in the third group took placebos. All of the men completed the trial. The researchers found that relatively small amounts of flaxseed lignan extract improved the subjects' cholesterol levels and ratios. In addition, the men experienced decreases in waist circumference, which is important for cardiovascular health.

Researchers from the University of Texas, the United Kingdom, and China analyzed twenty-eight studies on the effects of flaxseed interventions on blood lipids. They found that flaxseed interventions decreased both total cholesterol and LDL levels. Interestingly, reduced cholesterol levels were more prevalent in women, especially postmenopausal women, than men. No significant changes were observed in HDL, or "good" cholesterol, and triglyceride levels.

Irritable Bowel Syndrome

Researchers in the United Kingdom wanted to learn if flaxseeds would alleviate irritable bowel syndrome symptoms, such as bloating and constipation. They began by dividing forty subjects diagnosed with irritable bowel syndrome into three groups. The subjects in one group took two tablespoons of whole flaxseeds each day, the subjects in the second group took two tablespoons of ground flaxseeds each day, and the subjects in the third group ate their usual diets. After four weeks, thirty-one subjects were still in the trial, and the researchers learned that flaxseed supplementation significantly decreased the severity of the subjects' symptoms.

Prostate Health

As men age, they're at increased risk for experiencing benign prostatic hyperplasia, a condition in which the prostate gland is enlarged due to inflammation. This condition affects the lower urinary tract and causes a number of uncomfortable symptoms, such as the urgency to urinate and problems urinating. While there are treatments for this medical problem, they're not always effective, and they may have side effects. Sometimes surgery is the only feasible option. That's why researchers at the James R. Randall Research Center at the Archer Daniels Midland Company in Decatur, Illinois, and in China, tested the ability of flaxseeds to relieve the inflammation associated with this condition. The researchers divided eighty-seven Chinese men with benign prostatic hyperplasia into three groups. For four months, the men in two of the groups took different doses of flaxseed lignan supplements; the men in the third group took placebos. Seventy-eight men completed the trial. The researchers found that flaxseed lignan supplements relieved the symptoms associated with benign prostate hyperplasia and improved the men's quality of life. In fact, the flaxseed lignan supplements were about as effective as commonly prescribed prescription drugs.

The fiber in flaxseeds may interfere with the absorption of oral medications, so it's best not to consume flaxseeds at the same time you're taking medications or supplements.

Type 2 Diabetes

Researchers in India wanted to determine if flaxseeds would be useful for people with type 2 diabetes, who are not only affected by blood glucose levels but often also by high cholesterol levels. The researchers divided twenty-nine subjects with type 2 diabetes into two groups. For one month, the subjects in one group took 10 grams of flaxseed powder every day; the subjects in the second group received no supplementation. The researchers found that flaxseed supplementation decreased fasting blood glucose by 19.7 percent and lowered glycated hemoglobin, a measurement of the average blood sugar concentrations over a period of time, by 15.6 percent. Subjects also experienced reductions in total cholesterol, triglyceride, and LDL levels and increases in HDL, or "good" cholesterol, levels.

GARLIC

One of the oldest cultivated plants in the world, garlic is native to central Asia and has been used as a food and medicine for thousands of years. In fact, garlic was given to the slaves of ancient Egypt to enhance their strength and well-being. The Egyptians knew that healthier slaves could be more productive.

Garlic is a member of the allium family, which also includes chives, leeks, and onions. A variety of sulfur-containing compounds gives garlic its pungent odor and is responsible for many of garlic's health benefits. In addition, garlic contains an abundant array of nutrients, such as calcium, copper, manganese, phosphorus, selenium, tryptophan, and vitamins B_1, B_6, and C.

In terms of health benefits, garlic is probably best known for preventing cardiovascular disease by decreasing cholesterol and triglyceride levels and protecting blood cells and blood vessels against inflammation and oxidative stress. Garlic also lowers blood pressure and reduces the risk of blood clots. In addition, garlic has antibacterial and antiviral properties. And last but not least, there's evidence that garlic helps prevent cancer and may be useful in the treatment of cancer.

To obtain the most nutrients and health benefits from garlic, purchase fresh garlic that feels firm to the touch. While some stores sell packages of peeled garlic cloves, garlic is most often sold in bulbs that are formed by several small cloves. The bulb and cloves are covered with a very thin, paperlike skin that is white, off-white, or pinkish in color. At home, store garlic bulbs in a cool, dark place.

Garlic is available in a number of forms and may also be sold as a powder or as granules. In recent years, black garlic has gained increasing popularity and is available as a packaged product in some grocery stores or online. Black garlic is fermented, which transforms both the texture and taste, making it softer and sweeter. Many people find it far more palatable than regular garlic.

GARLIC	1 CLOVE
Calories	4
Fat	3%
Carbohydrates	85%
Protein	12%

Burn Infections

Researchers from Ahvaz Jundishapur University of Medical Sciences in Iran wondered whether giving burn victims fresh garlic would be useful in preventing infections. Patients suffering from burns have an increased risk for infection, particularly from the common bacterium *Pseudomonas aeruginosa*. The researchers divided 140 patients with burns into three groups according to the size of the burns. Each group was then subdivided into a treatment group and a control group. The members of the treatment groups received two crushed garlic cloves mixed into yogurt with their daily lunch; the members of the control groups received only yogurt. The researchers found that the patients with moderate burn injuries benefited from the addition of garlic to their diets; significantly fewer of them developed burn wound infections.

Cancer

In a small pilot study conducted at four different locations in the United States, researchers developed a urine test that shows that people who consume the greatest amounts of garlic have the lowest levels of potential cancer cells in their bodies. The research began with a small human study at Penn State University in University Park, Pennsylvania, and soon expanded to include other researchers. Altogether, their findings showed that people who consumed only 5 grams of garlic per day had the fewest markers for potential cancer cell growth. Since one garlic clove usually weighs between 1 and 5 grams, a relatively small amount of garlic appears to make a notable difference in preventing cancer.

Hoping to learn if garlic is useful in protecting against colorectal cancer, researchers at several locations in Australia conducted a systematic review of the literature. The researchers began by noting that colorectal cancer is the second leading cause of death in Australia. Therefore, finding foods that may play a role in preventing this type of cancer is very important. The researchers reviewed forty-three studies published over the previous ten years that examined the effects of garlic or garlic constitu-ents on colorectal cancer. Overall, the researchers found that a significant number of studies showed that people who eat greater amounts of garlic tend to have lower rates of colorectal cancer.

In a separate literature review conducted at three different loca-tions in Chengdu, China, researchers evaluated studies that linked the consumption of large amounts of allium vegetables to a reduced risk for gastric, or stomach, cancer. The review included twenty-one studies, with a total of 543,220 subjects. The researchers found that the subjects who consumed large amounts of allium vegetables had a lower risk for gastric cancer. When the researchers reviewed the studies on garlic alone, they obtained similar results.

Researchers at three different locations in Korea tested the ability of aged black garlic to prevent alcohol-induced liver injury in rats. They divided the rats into three groups. The control group was fed saline, or salt water, a second group was fed ethanol, and a third group was fed ethanol and aged black garlic. Ethanol is an alcohol that was used to induce liver damage. The study continued for four weeks. As expected, the ethanol caused liver damage to the rats in the second group. However, the rats that were given ethanol and aged black garlic had far less liver damage.

Cardiovascular Health

In a twelve-week study conducted at several locations in Korea, research-ers assessed the effects of aged garlic extract and regular exercise on thirty postmenopausal women. The women were divided into four intervention groups, and only two of the four groups exercised. The nonexercising group was composed of six women who were given a placebo and eight women who were given aged garlic extract. The group that exercised regularly was composed of eight women who were given a placebo and eight women who were given aged garlic extract. The researchers found that the women who took aged garlic extract or exercised regularly expe-rienced improvements in a number of factors that support cardiovascular health. For example, they had decreases in body weight, body fat, body mass index, and LDL, or "bad" cholesterol. The researchers noted that the effects of aged garlic extract appeared to be independent of the effects of exercise in postmenopausal women, so both aged garlic extract and regular exercise (used independently or together) are useful in support-ing cardiovascular health.

Researchers at the University of Adelaide in South Australia and Australia's National Institute of Integrative Medicine in Melbourne tested the use of different doses of aged garlic extract on seventy-nine subjects

Garlic may interact with the effectiveness of the blood-thinning medication warfarin, which helps prevent blood clots. If you're using warfarin, discuss the use of garlic with your medical provider.

with elevated and uncontrolled systolic (top number) blood pressure. For twelve weeks, the subjects took one of three different doses of aged garlic extract or a placebo. The subjects taking the high and medium doses of aged garlic extract had reductions in systolic blood pressure, leaving the researchers to conclude that aged garlic extract could be an effective component of treatment for uncontrolled high blood pressure.

Researchers from Shandong University in China reviewed twenty-six research studies that investigated the influence of garlic on blood lipid levels. They learned that in comparison with placebos, garlic effectively reduced total cholesterol and triglyceride levels. The effects of garlic were more dramatic in people who had high total cholesterol levels at the start of the study and used garlic for longer periods of time. According to the researchers, garlic didn't appear to influence other blood lipid levels, such as LDL and HDL, or "good" cholesterol.

Hip Osteoarthritis

Here's one final study on garlic, and this one examines the association between garlic consumption and hip osteoarthritis. United Kingdom researchers reviewed data from a large study of twins. Many of the subjects had no arthritis symptoms. Yet, using X-ray images, the researchers were able to see the extent of early osteoarthritis in the subjects' hips, knees, and spines. The researchers found that the subjects who consumed greater amounts of fruits and vegetables (especially members of the genus *Allium*, such as garlic) had less evidence of early osteoarthritis in the hip joint.

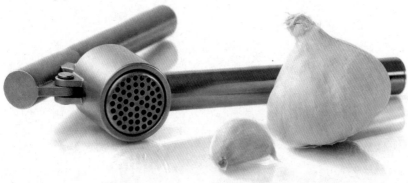

KALE

Like broccoli, Brussels sprouts, and cabbage, kale is a leafy green cruciferous vegetable that originated in the far western part of the Asian continent. Most likely, Celtic wanderers introduced kale to Europe around 600 BC. In the seventeenth century, English settlers brought kale to the United States.

The most common variety of kale is curly kale, which can be green or purple; this form of kale is so attractive, it's often used as a garnish. However, with its sweet and mild taste, not to mention its off-the-charts nutrition quotient, curly kale deserves a starring role, not a cameo appearance, on your dinner plate. The second most common type of kale is dinosaur, also called lacinato, kale. This distinctive form of dark green kale has tall, narrow leaves and a wrinkled texture. In general, the two types of kale can be successfully interchanged in most recipes.

Kale has a truly star-studded cast of nutrients. These include vitamins A, B_1, B_2, B_3, B_6, C, E, K, and folate and a variety of minerals, such as calcium, copper, iron, magnesium, manganese, phosphorus, and potassium. Kale is gaining attention because it's so rich in calcium, and the calcium in kale is absorbed by the body twice as well as calcium from dairy products. Kale is also an excellent source of fiber, omega-3 fatty acids, protein, and the essential amino acid tryptophan. In addition, kale is rich in two types of antioxidants: carotenoids and flavonoids. Yet, despite being such a nutrition heavyweight, kale is a very low-calorie food.

Having fully earned its rank as a superfood, kale has strong anti-inflammatory properties, supports cardiovascular health, and aggressively kills cancer cells. Some researchers have concluded that kale and other cruciferous vegetables are more potent cancer fighters when eaten raw. When chopped or chewed, the sulfur-containing compounds in kale, called glucosinolates, form isothiocyanates, which are known to prevent cancer. However, cooking can substantially reduce or destroy the isothiocyanates in kale. If you haven't tried raw kale before, there are two very palatable ways to incorporate it into your diet: blend it into a fruit smoothie or chop it into small pieces and use it in a marinated salad. After marinating in a dressing for about twenty minutes, raw kale leaves will soften. Alternatively, small pieces of fresh kale can be softened by "massaging" them with olive oil and lemon juice, and even bits of ripe avocado. To keep fresh kale from wilting, store it in a plastic bag in the refrigerator.

Cancer

At Roswell Park Cancer Institute in Buffalo, New York, researchers reviewed studies that linked the sulfur-containing compounds in kale and other cruciferous vegetables to the prevention of bladder cancer. However, the studies, which included both laboratory research and research on living subjects, had inconsistent results. The researchers wondered if this occurred because the vegetables were sometimes cooked, which may reduce or destroy the amounts of isothiocyanates, the by-products of the sulfur-containing compounds in kale that deter cancer growth. In a hospital-based study, the researchers examined the intake of raw and cooked kale and other cruciferous vegetables in 275 people with bladder cancer and 825 randomly selected people who were being treated for conditions other than cancer. The researchers found a strong statistical association: the subjects who ate the greatest amounts of raw cruciferous vegetables had the lowest risk of bladder cancer.

Researchers from the Harvard School of Public Health in Boston and the University of California, San Francisco, observed that cruciferous vegetables such as kale, as well as tomato sauce and legumes, decrease the risk of advanced prostate cancer in men. Therefore, the researchers decided to investigate whether the intake of cruciferous vegetables, tomato

KALE	1 CUP
Calories	34
Fat	12%
Carbohydrates	71%
Protein	17%

THYROID PROBLEMS?

Like all cruciferous vegetables, kale contains goitrogens, compounds that may interfere with the functioning of the thyroid gland. The amount of goitrogens is reduced when kale is steamed, cooked, or fermented. Those who have concerns about thyroid health should consult with their doctors before consuming kale, especially in large quantities. People with thyroid problems may want to avoid raw kale and limit their overall intake, eating cooked kale only occasionally.

sauce, and legumes would affect men who had already been diagnosed with nonmetastatic (nonspreading) prostate cancer. Over the course of five years, the researchers studied 1,560 men. When compared to the men who ate the smallest amounts of the studied foods, the men who ate the greatest amounts had a statistically significant 59 percent decrease in their risk of cancer progression. The researchers concluded that prostate cancer was considerably less likely to spread in the men who consumed cruciferous vegetables after diagnosis.

In a similar study, researchers at the Linus Pauling Institute at Oregon State University in Corvallis reviewed many studies on the ability of cruciferous vegetables to lower the risk of cancer in humans. The researchers found good evidence that the consumption of cruciferous vegetables reduces the risk of breast, colorectal, lung, and prostate cancer. They also noted that kale and other cruciferous vegetables may lower the risk of pancreatic cancer, although the evidence for this wasn't as strong.

Researchers from several institutions in Quebec, Canada, including the Ministry of Agriculture, Sainte-Justine University Hospital Center, and the University of Quebec, conducted laboratory tests to examine the anticancer properties of thirty-four vegetables against brain, breast, kidney, lung, pancreas, prostate, and stomach cancer cells. The researchers found that kale had some of the strongest anticancer properties and can help kill cancer cells that develop in the body, in addition to preventing cancer cells from growing. Interestingly, the researchers noted that common vegetables, such as carrots, potatoes, and tomatoes, appeared to have little, if any, effect against cancer growth.

Researchers at the Metametrix Institute in Duluth, Georgia, were aware that some people consume no, or only small amounts of, cruciferous vegetables either because they don't like these foods or the foods aren't regularly available. So the researchers decided to test a supplement containing dried organic kale and Brussels sprouts to determine whether supplement use could raise a marker for anticancer activity in estrogen-sensitive tissues, such as those found in the breasts of premenopausal women. Twenty-three women originally agreed to participate in the study. Thirteen women between the ages of thirty-four and forty-seven completed the ninety-day trial. Twice daily, they took capsules that contained 300 milligrams of dried organic kale and 300 milligrams of dried organic Brussels sprouts, a total daily intake of 3.6 grams of dried whole vegetables equal to about 36 grams of fresh vegetables. The results of this trial were rather dramatic, with eleven of the thirteen subjects demonstrating strongly positive increases in the marker for anticancer activity.

Cardiovascular Health

At the Shanghai Cancer Institute in China, researchers wanted to learn how the consumption of cruciferous vegetables, noncruciferous vegetables, total vegetables, and fruit affected the incidence of morbidity, or death, in a population. They analyzed the findings from two population-based studies involving 134,796 Chinese adults. At the time of enrollment, the average age of the subjects in one study was fifty-three, and in the other study it was fifty-five. The women had an average follow-up of 10.2 years, during which time there were 3,442 deaths. The men had an average follow-up of 4.6 years, during which time there were 1,951 deaths. The researchers found that an increased consumption of total vegetables, especially cruciferous vegetables such as kale, and fruit significantly reduced overall mortality, primarily because there were fewer deaths from cardiovascular disease.

Researchers at the United States Department of Agriculture's West Regional Research Center in Albany, California, determined that steamed leafy vegetables, such as kale, lower the risk of cardiovascular disease and cancer when consumed regularly. One reason is because steaming kale increases its ability to bind with bile acids in the digestive tract. After the kale and bile acids are bound, they're eliminated from the body in the stool. When this occurs, the liver must replace the lost bile acids from the body's supply of cholesterol. That process, in turn, lowers cholesterol levels. Raw kale is also able to bind with bile acids; however, the process is far more effective when the kale has been steamed. The researchers compared kale's ability to bind with bile acids to that of cholestyramine, a medication that also lowers cholesterol by binding with bile acids. Of all the vegetables tested, kale was the most efficient in binding with bile acids. Compared to cholestyramine, kale was 13 percent as effective in binding with bile acids. So although the medication performed better, kale did have notable results.

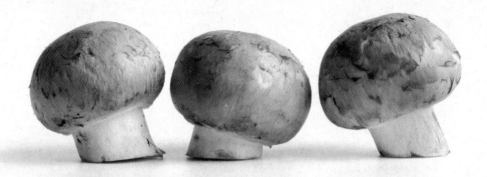

MUSHROOMS

or centuries, mushrooms have played a key role in the therapeutic practices of traditional Eastern healers. Still, until fairly recent times, the Western world appeared to be unaware of the medicinal powers of mushrooms.

Although they're often thought to be vegetables, mushrooms are actually fungi. Rich in nutrients, such as proteins, vitamins, and minerals, mushrooms have the ability to heal and repair cells. In addition, they're very low in calories and carbohydrates, high in fiber and B vitamins, and abundant in niacin, riboflavin, and selenium.

People at risk for cardiovascular problems are encouraged to eat foods that are rich in potassium, a mineral that lowers blood pressure and reduces the risk of stroke. Daily consumption of mushrooms, which are an outstanding source of potassium, can prevent a shortage of this important mineral. Though it may be hard to believe, just one portobello mushroom, which can be used as a meat substitute, has more potassium than a glass of orange juice or a banana, both of which are touted as being high in potassium.

Mushrooms are wonderfully varied and provide a range of health benefits. Even the most common mushroom sold in the world, the everyday button mushroom, makes an uncommon contribution to human health: button mushrooms are known to kill cancer cells. Fresh or canned button mushrooms are readily available in supermarkets nationwide, and they boast very high levels of B vitamins along with potassium.

Shiitake mushrooms, which are gaining in popularity, have brown, slightly convex caps and a rich, smoky flavor. They're noted for supporting cardiovascular health and immune function and for destroying cancer cells. Exceedingly rich in iron, shiitake mushrooms are also a good source of the minerals copper, manganese, phosphorus, potassium, selenium, and zinc. In addition, shiitake mushrooms are an excellent source of vitamins B_2, B_5, and B_6.

MUSHROOMS	1 CUP, SLICED
Calories	15
Fat	13%
Carbohydrates	52%
Protein	35%

Other common mushrooms include brown, or cremini, mushrooms, which are meaty and earthy, and portobello mushrooms, which are simply fully grown brown mushrooms. Another variety that can sometimes be found in supermarkets, oyster mushrooms have a mild, delicate flavor.

Cancer

In research involving mice, scientists from the Beckman Research Institute at City of Hope in Duarte, California, tested the effects of white button mushroom extract on prostate cancer cells. The researchers found that within seventy-two hours of treatment, the extract inhibited the growth of prostate cancer cells; when more extract was used, fewer cancer cells grew. Similarly, white button mushroom extract decreased the size of prostate cancer tumors in mice and slowed the spreading of prostate cancer cells.

Researchers from the University of Western Australia and two locations in China studied the dietary intake of mushrooms and green tea in over one thousand women in Southeast China. The subjects were between the ages of twenty and eighty-seven and were newly diagnosed with breast cancer. The researchers conducted in-person interviews to learn about the subjects' intake of mushrooms and green tea. They found that the women who ate the most fresh or dried mushrooms had a significantly lower risk of breast cancer. The most commonly consumed fresh mushrooms were button mushrooms. This reduced risk was seen in both premenopausal and postmenopausal women. In addition, the subjects who drank green tea had a reduced risk for breast cancer.

A report from the University of Pennsylvania School of Veterinary Medicine describes how a compound derived from a common mushroom promises to be an effective alternative or complementary treatment for dogs who have cancer. Two researchers studied dogs with hemangiosarcoma, an aggressive and invasive cancer that forms in blood cells and affects the spleen. The dogs were treated with different doses of a compound found in *Coriolus versicolor* (also called yunzhi or turkey tail mushrooms), which are used in Traditional Chinese Medicine. Some of the dogs treated with the mushroom compound had the longest survival times ever reported for dogs with hemangiosarcoma. Normally, dogs with this medical problem live only a few months following diagnosis, but some of the treated dogs lived more than one year after diagnosis. The dogs on the highest dose lived the longest. The researchers suggested that the mushroom formula may also be effective in treating people with cancer.

Dental Health

Researchers from Italy, London, Sweden, and the Netherlands joined together to test the antimicrobial and antiplaque properties of shiitake mushroom extract. Ninety men and women were recruited for the study and were divided into three groups of thirty. For twelve days, the volunteers in each group rinsed their mouths twice daily with either shiitake mushroom extract, Listerine mouthwash, or water (the placebo). The researchers found that the shiitake mushroom extract was significantly better at reducing dental plaque than water but wasn't significantly better than Listerine. When it came to reducing gum inflammation, however, the shiitake mushroom extract was significantly better than both water and Listerine, leaving the researchers to conclude that the extract can be beneficial in preventing common dental problems.

High Cholesterol and Type 2 Diabetes

Researchers from Australia and South Korea investigated the effects of feeding white button mushroom powder to rats with laboratory-induced type 2 diabetes or elevated cholesterol levels. When compared to rats with type 2 diabetes that didn't receive treatment, the rats consuming the supplemental powder for three weeks had significant decreases in blood glucose (sugar) levels and triglyceride concentrations. In addition, the rats with elevated levels of cholesterol that consumed the supplemental powder for four weeks had significant decreases in total cholesterol levels.

Memory

Researchers in Japan noted that memory problems, especially among older people, are a serious social and public health concern. Since it's known that *Hericium erinaceus* (more commonly referred to as hedgehog mushrooms) heal the nervous system, the researchers wanted to learn if this mushroom could improve memory. They studied a group of thirty men and women between the ages of fifty and eighty who had been diagnosed with mild memory impairment. Half of the subjects were randomly placed in a mushroom treatment group, and the other half received a placebo. The treatment continued for sixteen weeks. The researchers observed that the people taking the mushroom supplementation showed significant improvements in memory at that point. However, the subjects' memory scores markedly decreased four weeks after supplementation was discontinued, leaving the researchers to conclude that memory improvement was dependent upon sustained supplementation.

Weight Loss

Researchers at the Johns Hopkins Bloomberg School of Public Health in Baltimore, Maryland, postulated that people could lose weight if they substituted white button mushrooms for ground beef. To test their theory, the researchers recruited men and women to eat lunches on four consecutive weekdays during two consecutive weeks at the school's Center for Human Nutrition. The volunteers ate four lunches in which white button mushrooms were used instead of ground beef and four lunches that included ground beef but not mushrooms. Eighteen men and thirty-six women completed the study and found the mushrooms to be a palatable and satisfying replacement for beef. As a result, the researchers concluded that white button mushrooms could be one of a number of low-calorie and low-fat meat replacements. The researchers noted that if people made such a substitution only once per week, they could lose five pounds in one year.

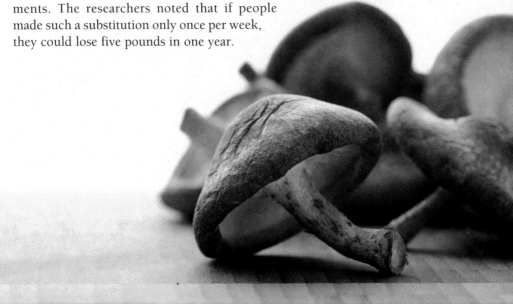

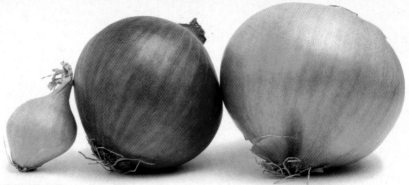

ONIONS

Like the superfood garlic, onions belong to the allium family and are rich in sulfur-containing compounds that give them their pungent aroma. Although onions, especially raw onions, may be a little strong for some tastes, they're also powerfully nutritious. They contain fiber, protein, and a range of vitamins, such as B_6, C, and folic acid. In addition, onions are rich in minerals, including calcium, iron, magnesium, manganese, phosphorous, and potassium.

Like all vegetables, onions are abundant in antioxidants, which are also called phytochemicals; they're especially rich in quercetin, a flavonoid that helps slow damage to the body's cells. Interestingly, most of the flavonoid in onions is concentrated in the outer layers of the flesh, so removing these layers eliminates much of this very important antioxidant.

Native to Asia and the Middle East, onions have been cultivated for more than five thousand years. The ancient Egyptians regarded them with great awe and put them in the tombs of the pharaohs, believing the onions were necessary in the great leaders' afterlives. Egyptians also paid workers with onions, so perhaps this humble vegetable played a mighty role in building the Egyptian empire.

By the sixth century, residents of India considered onions to have medicinal properties, and onions grew in popularity. In fact, since onions were relatively inexpensive, they were even used widely in communities with limited resources. Onions also were popular in Europe during the Middle Ages, and Christopher Columbus brought onions to the West

ONIONS	1 CUP, CHOPPED
Calories	67
Fat	2%
Carbohydrates	92%
Protein	6%

Indies. Today, the leading producers of onions are the United States, China, India, Russia, and Spain.

When shopping, choose onions that are clean and firm. Try to avoid onions that are sprouting or have soft spots. At home, it's best to store whole onions at room temperature. Green onions, also known as scallions, or cut onions should be stored in the refrigerator.

Bone Health

Researchers from the Department of Family Medicine at the Medical University of South Carolina in Charleston examined the association between onion consumption and bone density in women. Previous research involving animal studies had suggested that flavonoids, including quercetin, in onions appear to promote bone growth and decrease the rate of bone breakdown. Researchers at the University of Bern, Switzerland, identified a key bioactive compound, a peptide called GPCS, in onions that may help prevent osteoporosis. In the human study, the subjects were perimenopausal and postmenopausal non-Hispanic white women age fifty and older. The researchers divided the 507 women into four groups, according to how frequently they consumed onions: once a month or less, twice a month to twice a week, three to six times a week, and once a day or more. The researchers found that the subjects who ate the most onions had the highest bone density. In fact, when compared to women who ate no onions, the women who ate the most onions reduced their risk of hip fractures by more than 20 percent.

Cancer

Researchers at multiple locations in Taiwan analyzed the food intake of 343 patients with squamous cell cancer of the esophagus and compared them to 755 comparable but cancer-free subjects. After comprehensively studying the subjects' food intake, the researchers found strong evidence that raw onions were among the foods that lowered the risk of developing this disease.

At the Medical Sciences Center at the University of Wisconsin-Madison, researchers investigated the anticancer properties of fisetin, a flavonoid found in onions and other foods. As a result of their laboratory studies, the researchers determined that fisetin has the ability to stop the growth of prostate cancer cells, whereas it has only a minimal effect on normal cells. They noted that fisetin may be developed as an agent to fight prostate cancer.

Flavonoids are abundant in onions, but black tea is a better-known source. Researchers from the United Kingdom, the Republic of Ireland, and the University of Ottawa in Canada studied the intake of flavonoids obtained from sources other than tea. As a result of research involving 264 people with colorectal cancer and 408 healthy, cancer-free people, the scientists found that flavonoids obtained from non-tea sources, such as onions, are associated with a reduced risk of developing colon cancer but not rectal cancer.

Cardiovascular Health

Researchers from the United Kingdom and Spain examined the compounds that enter the blood after the consumption and digestion of foods that contain quercetin. Their research led them to determine that foods with quercetin help prevent the chronic inflammation that may lead to cardiovascular disease.

The American Heart Association has estimated that 74.5 million Americans have hypertension or high blood pressure, and about 25 percent of the population has prehypertension. Acknowledging the implications for public health, researchers from the Central Washington University in Ellensburg, Washington, and the University of Utah in Salt Lake City studied the effects of quercetin, which is abundant in onions and has been proven to lower blood pressure in both animals and humans. In their own studies involving humans, the researchers found that quercetin supplementation for twenty-eight days lowered blood pressure in people with hypertension but not in people with prehypertension.

Influenza

Researchers from the University of South Carolina in Columbia and Clemson University in South Carolina were aware that exercise stress has been associated with an increased risk for upper respiratory tract infections. They wanted to learn if quercetin could decrease this risk and designed an animal study to investigate. The study involved mice, which were divided into four groups. Two groups of mice exercised on a treadmill on three consecutive days, and only one of the exercise groups was given quercetin. The mice in the other two groups didn't exercise, and only one of the sedentary groups was given quercetin. The researchers found that the mice that ran but didn't receive quercetin were at increased risk for infection; however, quercetin lowered the risk of infection in the second group of running mice. In addition, the mice that ran developed the flu sooner than those that didn't. Interestingly, the rate of illness in the mice that exercised and took quercetin was about the same as the rate in the mice that didn't exercise. The researchers suggested that quercetin supplementation minimized the negative effects of stressful exercise. Onions are a natural source of quercetin, but people who have problems digesting raw or cooked onions may wish to consider taking quercetin supplements to avoid respiratory infections and other health problems.

Prostate Health

Benign prostate hyperplasia, or enlargement of the prostate gland, is a very common and uncomfortable problem that occurs most often in older men. An enlarged prostate makes it more difficult for men to urinate. In addition, men who are affected by this condition may need to awaken several times during the night to urinate, which disrupts sleep. That's why researchers from Italy and France tested the ability of onions (and garlic) to provide some relief from this disorder. Their study included 1,369 men with enlarged prostate glands and 1,451 comparable men without this problem. The researchers found that the men who ate the most onions (and garlic) were least likely to have this medical condition.

Protruding Scars

Researchers from several different surgical departments at Khon Kaen University in Thailand observed that protruding scars can present significant problems for patients, and prominent scars may cause ongoing physical and emotional side effects. For example, protruding scars may itch or interfere with mobility. So the researchers decided to investigate how scars responded to treatment with a gel made from onion extract and medical-grade silicone. Sixty surgery patients were included in the double-blind study, and neither the researchers nor the patients knew who was treated with the onion-based gel or a placebo product. The treatments continued twice each day for twelve weeks, and fifty-four patients completed the study. The researchers found that the men and women using the onion gel experienced less itching and pain than those using the placebo. The treated scars also had less pigmentation, or dark coloring, making them less noticeable than the scars treated with placebo. In addition, the onion gel showed some other positive attributes: it had no side effects and could easily be removed.

SEA VEGETABLES

People have consumed sea vegetables, also known as seaweed, for thousands of years. In fact, archaeological evidence shows that the Japanese have been eating sea vegetables for more than ten thousand years. Sea vegetables have long been a dietary staple not only in Japan but also in other Asian countries, such as Korea and Vietnam, and a number of other maritime countries, such as Iceland, Ireland, New Zealand, and Scotland.

Despite having almost no calories, sea vegetables pack a powerful nutrient punch. They have excellent amounts of vitamin K and iodine, very good amounts of folate and magnesium, and good amounts of calcium, iron, pantothenic acid, riboflavin, tryptophan, and vitamins C and E. They also contain sulfated polysaccharides, also known as fucoidans, which fight inflammation, viral infections, and cardiovascular disease.

There are countless varieties of sea vegetables, which are typically classified by color: brown, green, or red. In the kitchen, sea vegetables can be used to make sushi, or they can be added to casseroles, salads, soups, stir-fries, and many other dishes. Some commonly available sea vegetables include arame, dulse, nori, and wakame.

Wiry in appearance, arame is sweet and mild and makes a tasty addition to salads and cooked vegetables. Dulse is soft and chewy, and many people enjoy eating this sea vegetable raw; in fact, dulse is often sold as flakes that can be conveniently sprinkled atop salads and many other dishes. Nori is the familiar green sea vegetable that is formed into sheets and used to make sushi. Wakame, which is sold in sheets or strips, is delightful in miso soup. Except for nori and sea vegetables that are sold as ready-to-sprinkle flakes, most sea vegetables should be soaked in water before using; check the label for directions.

Cancer

Researchers in Malaysia compared the ability of red sea vegetables and tamoxifen, a medication used to treat breast cancer, to kill breast cancer cells in rats. The researchers found that the sea vegetables prevented the spread of breast cancer more effectively than the tamoxifen. In addition, tamoxifen is known to have several negative side effects, but the sea vegetables have none.

SEA VEGETABLES	1 CUP
Calories	30
Fat	5%
Carbohydrates	74%
Protein	21%

In a study conducted at Japan's Red Cross Kyoto Daiichi Hospital, researchers investigated the effects of eating certain fruits and vegetables on colorectal cancer risk. Based on the colonoscopy results and dietary information from 893 subjects, the researchers found that the women who ate larger amounts of sea vegetables had more than 75 percent fewer incidences of colorectal cancer; however, the same results weren't seen in the male subjects.

Researchers from the Gyeongsang National University in South Korea and Rutgers University in New Jersey examined the ability of fucoidan, which is derived from brown sea vegetables, to stop or slow the progression of aggressive human lung cancer cells that are highly likely to spread. Because fucoidan decreased the activity of these cells, the researchers concluded that fucoidan could be considered a therapeutic agent against this type of deadly cancer. Notably, the fucoidan didn't harm normal cells, which is significant because standard chemotherapy treatment kills both healthy and cancerous cells.

Herpes Virus

Researchers in Australia and at the University of Chicago explained that certain types of herpes virus are far less common in Japanese women than in American women, possibly because Japanese women eat far more sea vegetables. So the researchers recruited and treated fifteen subjects with active cases of herpes virus, including chicken pox, cold sores, genital herpes, mononucleosis, and shingles. They also treated six people with latent herpes infections. The subjects were given supplements containing wakame, one of the most commonly eaten sea vegetables in Japan, and the dosages approximated the daily intake of sea vegetables in Japan. The subjects were treated from one to twenty-four months, and the researchers found that the sea vegetable supplements improved healing, inhibited outbreaks in people with active infections, and reduced pain levels in some subjects. While being treated with sea vegetables,

If cooking with sea vegetables seems a little daunting, look for the various sea vegetable flakes that are sold in small shaker bottles (like the ones that contain spices). Nothing could be easier than shaking the contents right onto your food to benefit from the many nutrients in sea vegetables.

those with latent infections remained asymptomatic. In addition to conducting this human study, the researchers studied cell cultures in their laboratories, where they found that sea vegetables increased the growth of infection-fighting T cells.

Knee Osteoarthritis

Researchers in Australia tested a brand of sea vegetable extract called Maritech in twelve men and women who had a confirmed diagnosis of knee osteoarthritis and experienced pain, stiffness, and difficulty with physical activity. The subjects were assigned to take daily doses of either 100 or 1,000 milligrams of Maritech. Eleven subjects completed the full twelve-week study, and one subject completed ten weeks of the study. At the end of the study, the researchers concluded that Maritech effectively decreased the subjects' symptoms, with the higher dose being more effective. The 1,000-milligram dose reduced symptoms by 52 percent, whereas the 100-milligram dose reduced symptoms by 18 percent.

In another study, researchers from three locations in Minnesota recruited twenty-two subjects between the ages of thirty-five and seventy-five with moderate to severe knee osteoarthritis. For twelve weeks, the subjects took either a supplement manufactured from red sea vegetables or a placebo. After two weeks, the subjects were told to reduce their use of nonsteroidal anti-inflammatory drugs (NSAIDs), a common arthritis treatment, by about half; after four weeks, they were told to stop using the NSAIDs altogether. Instead, the subjects were instructed to manage their pain with acetaminophen. Fourteen of the subjects completed the entire trial, with more subjects dropping out of the placebo group because they were unable to tolerate their knee pain. The acetaminophen didn't provide sufficient pain relief; however, the subjects who were also taking the sea vegetable supplement had an increased ability to walk, and they moved about with greater ease. Moreover, they were able to reduce the amount of NSAIDs they used to control their knee pain.

Mild Acne

Researchers from Italy and the United Kingdom investigated whether a topical cream containing sea vegetables and zinc would be useful for sixty men who were treated for mild acne at a dermatological clinic in Rome. The men were treated with either the sea vegetable cream or with a cream without the added sea vegetables and zinc. For eight weeks, the men used the cream twice daily. After just two weeks, the researchers noted significant reductions in mild acne in the men using the sea vegetable cream. By the end of the trial, the men in both groups had less acne; however, the men using the sea vegetable cream had significantly better improvement. The sea vegetable cream effectively cleared blackheads, whiteheads, and lesions.

Weight Loss

Researchers at the University of Copenhagen in Frederiksberg, Denmark, investigated the ability of sea vegetable supplementation combined with a calorie-restricted diet to help obese people lose weight. Ninety-six subjects were divided into two groups: one group ate a calorie-restricted diet and took a supplement derived from sea vegetables, and the other group ate a calorie-restricted diet and took a placebo. The subjects were directed to take the supplement or placebo three times per day before meals for twelve weeks. When the study concluded, the researchers found that the subjects taking the sea vegetable supplement experienced more weight loss, primarily from a reduction in body fat. However, the researchers determined that the subjects in the placebo group had greater decreases in systolic and diastolic blood pressure, which prompted them to note that it's important to know the amount of sodium in supplements. High sodium intake can raise blood pressure.

In the United Kingdom, researchers tested the effects of a sea vegetable–based supplement on sixty-nine men and women. For seven days, some of the subjects took a sea vegetable supplement before meals, and the other subjects consumed a low-fat meal replacement powder before meals. Then the groups switched, with all subjects consuming the alternate product. Sixty-eight subjects were considered in the final analysis, in which the researchers found that the subjects had a lower daily intake of calories when taking the sea vegetable supplement.

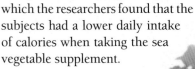

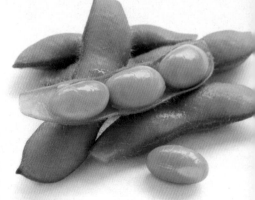

SOYBEANS

Like many other superfoods, soybeans have ancient roots. They have been cultivated in China for thousands of years and became a popular food in Japan and Korea well over a thousand years ago. Today much of the world depends on soybeans and other legumes as excellent sources of protein.

Soybeans are the seeds of the soybean plant, and like other legumes, they're commonly sold dried and are rehydrated during soaking and cooking. Store the dried beans in a tightly closed container for up to one year. Ready-to-use soybeans are available in cans. Soy nuts, a satisfying and crunchy snack, are not nuts at all but baked soybeans.

Nothing beats fresh soybeans, if you can find them. Some supermarkets and Asian groceries now sell fresh, immature soybeans, which are bright green; when they're cooked, they become an even brighter green. Fresh soybeans are often sold under the name "edamame," a general term used for soybeans that may or may not still be in the pod and are either raw or cooked. Fresh edamame should be stored in the refrigerator and eaten within one or two days; frozen edamame should be stored in the freezer and eaten within two months.

Beyond the dried, canned, and fresh versions of the bean, there are many other varieties of healthful soybean-based foods available. Tofu is a highly digestible form of soy. Sold in tubs or aseptic boxes, tofu is available in several different grades, from soft to extra-firm, and can be used in countless dishes, from stir-fries to creamy pies. Tempeh is made from fermented whole soybeans and is sold in blocks or cakes; it's a popular meat substitute. And finally, soy milk is an endlessly versatile alternative to cow's milk and is available just about everywhere.

In addition to being an outstanding source of protein, soybeans contain isoflavones, which are natural phytoestrogens and antioxidants. They're also an excellent source of fiber, omega-3 fatty acids, vitamins B_2 and K, and the minerals copper, iron, magnesium, manganese, and phosphorus. Soybeans are also rich in molybdenum, an essential element in human nutrition, and tryptophan, an important amino acid.

These abundant stores of nutrition translate into many healthful effects when people eat soy foods. For example, soybeans support cardio-

SOYBEANS	1 CUP
Calories	376
Fat	39%
Carbohydrates	31%
Protein	30%

vascular and bone health. They also help prevent cancer and calm menopausal symptoms, such as hot flashes. And because soybeans are a rich source of dietary fiber and protein, they're a valuable addition to the diets of people who have type 2 diabetes or need to lose weight.

Bone Health

Researchers from the Philippines and several locations in South Korea wanted to investigate the effects of soybeans on bone health. To do so, they designed a laboratory study involving rats. The researchers gave different concentrations of ungerminated and germinated soybeans to young male rats to see whether the soybeans promoted bone growth. The researchers divided forty-nine rats into seven groups and put them on different diets. Three groups of rats were fed varying amounts of ungerminated soybean powder, three groups were fed varying amounts of germinated soybean powder, and one group was fed no soybean powder. After ten weeks, the researchers found that the rats that were fed either type of soybean powder experienced increases in bone strength.

Researchers from three different universities in China reviewed nine studies involving soy isoflavone, an antioxidant and estrogenic compound abundant in soy foods, and its ability to stimulate bone formation and prevent bone depletion. The studies, which represented findings from 432 human subjects who were given isoflavone supplements, supported the use of soybeans to improve bone health. Moreover, the researchers found that supplementation was beneficial even in small amounts (less than 90 milligrams daily) and when used for less than twelve weeks, a somewhat brief intervention.

Cancer

Soybean meal is a by-product that's left when oil is extracted from soybean seeds. In laboratory tests, researchers at the University of Arkansas in Fayetteville evaluated the effects of soybean meal on colon, liver, and lung cancer cells. They found that soybean meal significantly inhibited the growth of 73 percent of colon cancer cells, 70 percent of liver cancer cells, and 68 percent of lung cancer cells. Higher concentrations of soybean meal inhibited the growth of even more cancer cells.

Researchers at Vanderbilt University Medical Center in Nashville, Tennessee, identified 444 women with lung cancer from the Shanghai Women's Health Study. (Worldwide, lung cancer is a leading cause of death in women.) The researchers assessed the women's intake of soy foods at three separate times: before their diagnosis, at the beginning of the study, and two years later. During the follow-up period, 318 of the women died. Despite the high mortality rate, the researchers were able to learn that the women who had a greater intake of soy foods before their diagnosis had better overall survival rates. Twelve months after diagnosis, 60 percent of those who ate the most soy and 50 percent of those who ate the least soy were still alive. Consuming about 4 ounces of tofu per day was effective in reducing risk; there was no additional survival benefit from consuming larger amounts of soy.

Cardiovascular Health

Researchers in Tokyo, Japan, reviewed the results of eleven clinical studies that linked the consumption of soybeans and reduced total cholesterol levels. According to these studies, eating soybeans significantly lowered levels of total cholesterol and LDL, or "bad" cholesterol. However, soybeans appeared to have no effect on HDL, or "good" cholesterol, or triglyceride levels. Reductions in LDL cholesterol were greater in people with elevated cholesterol levels than in people with normal cholesterol levels.

Another study, led by researchers from the Department of Epidemiology at Tulane University School of Public Health and Tropical Medicine in New Orleans, Louisiana, explored the connection between soybean protein and cardiovascular health. Researchers compared how 40 grams of soybean protein supplement per day, 40 grams of milk protein supplement per day, and 40 grams of complex carbohydrate (placebo) per day improved a number of markers of cardiovascular health. For eight weeks, 102 men and women, with an average age of forty-six, were assigned to take either the soybean protein, milk protein, or complex carbohydrate supplement. The researchers found that the subjects taking the soybean protein supplement had lower levels of certain markers, such as E-selectin and leptin, that impair cardiovascular health. By lowering those markers, soybeans support cardiovascular health.

CHOOSE ORGANIC SOY PRODUCTS

Savvy consumers often seek out organic foods, especially fresh produce, to avoid pesticides. In the case of soy foods, it's important to buy organic because the vast majority of soybeans are genetically modified. So look for soy products that are labeled organic or "non-GMO." (GMO is an acronym for "genetically modified organism.")

Hot Flashes

Researchers at Beth Israel Deaconess Medical Center in Boston wanted to learn if a compound obtained from soybeans would be useful for treating hot flashes, which are caused by declining estrogen levels, in menopausal women. The researchers recruited women between the ages of thirty-eight and sixty who experienced between four and fourteen hot flashes per day. The subjects were divided into three groups: two groups took two different doses of a soybean supplement daily, and the third group took a placebo. The researchers found that when compared to the women taking the placebo, the women in both treatment groups experienced a significant reduction in the number of hot flashes per day.

In another study, researchers from the National Institute of Health and Nutrition in Tokyo, Japan, and three universities in the United States evaluated seventeen trials involving the use of soybean products to treat hot flashes. The researchers found that subjects who consumed two daily servings of soy or took soy supplements for six weeks to twelve months had less frequent and less severe hot flashes. In fact, the frequency of hot flashes was reduced by an average of 20 percent and the severity by an average of 26 percent. In the studies that continued for longer periods, the decrease in hot flash frequency was about three times greater than in the studies that lasted for shorter periods, suggesting that soy more effectively controls hot flashes when it's eaten regularly over time.

Memory

Researchers from different locations in Japan tested the ability of a soybean-derived supplement to improve memory in seventy-eight subjects between the ages of fifty and sixty-nine who had memory complaints. The subjects were put into three groups: two groups took different doses of the supplement, and the third group took a placebo. The researchers found that the soybean-derived supplements improved memory; the improvements were about the same for the lower and higher supplement doses.

TURMERIC

Native to Indonesia and southern India, turmeric is a plant related to ginger that has been harvested for thousands of years. Arab traders introduced turmeric to Europe during the thirteenth century, but it wasn't until relatively recent times that turmeric gained popularity in many Western countries. Today, turmeric is grown primarily in China, Haiti, Indonesia, India, Jamaica, the Philippines, and Taiwan.

Parts of the turmeric plant are dried and ground into a powder to produce the spice that's used to make curry powder and yellow mustard. Turmeric has a peppery flavor and an aroma that's reminiscent of both orange and ginger. A deep yellow-orange in color, turmeric also is used as a textile dye.

Most significant in terms of its inclusion as a superfood is the fact that turmeric is also used as a healing remedy, especially for treating conditions associated with inflammation. The yellow or orange pigment in turmeric is known as curcumin, which is believed to contain turmeric's healing powers.

Aside from calming inflammation, the spice is also useful for a vast variety of medical conditions. These include appetite loss, arthritis, cancer, cardiovascular problems, colds, dementia, depression, diarrhea, fever, gallbladder disorders, gas, heartburn, jaundice, lung infections, menstrual problems, stomach pain, water retention, and worms. When applied directly to the skin, turmeric helps to heal bruises, infected wounds, inflammatory skin conditions, leech bites, and ringworm.

A report published in the *International Journal of Clinical Medicine* described just how effective turmeric can be in supporting multiple medical conditions. The report was written by and recounts the experiences of a sixty-one-year-old physician who was born and raised in southern India but has lived in the United States for more than thirty years. After eating curry, a popular Indian dish containing turmeric, every day for over fifty years, the doctor decided the dish was causing his frequent gastrointestinal disturbances. So he stopped eating it. About three months later, he developed pain and a burning sensation in his legs and feet. The pain

TURMERIC	1 TEASPOON
Calories	8
Fat	23%
Carbohydrates	70%
Protein	7%

persisted for six years. During this time, when he did eat turmeric, his pain improved, though only temporarily. He also began having memory problems, and his prostate-specific antigen (PSA) level, a measure of potential prostate cancer, increased. The physician decided to reintroduce a curry dish containing turmeric into his daily diet. After he ate it twice daily for about a week, his pain was manageable and his memory improved. After about nine weeks, his memory was restored and his PSA levels decreased.

Arthritis

Researchers at Siriraj Hospital in Bangkok, Thailand, divided 107 people with knee osteoarthritis into two groups. For six weeks, the subjects in the first group took 2 grams of turmeric per day, and the subjects in the second group took 800 milligrams of ibuprofen, an over-the-counter medication that reduces inflammation, per day. The researchers, who were unaware which treatment each subject was receiving, assessed their levels of improvement every two weeks for six weeks. Forty-five subjects in the turmeric group and forty-six subjects in the ibuprofen group completed the trial. The researchers found that the subjects in both groups experienced improvements, and most of the subjects were similarly satisfied with the treatments, rating themselves moderately to highly satisfied.

Another study on using turmeric for knee osteoarthritis was conducted by researchers at St. John's Medical College in Bangalore, India. The 120 subjects, who had all been diagnosed with knee osteoarthritis and had reported having pain for at least six months, were randomly assigned to one of four groups. The subjects in one group took a placebo; the subjects in a second group took 1,000 milligrams of turmeric per day; the subjects in a third group took 1,500 milligrams of glucosamine sulfate, a well-known supplement used for osteoarthritis, per day; and the subjects in the fourth group took both 1,000 milligrams of turmeric and 1,500 milligrams of glucosamine sulfate per day. All of the treatments were given in two divided doses. At the end of forty-two days, the subjects in all of the treatment groups experienced some degree of improvement. The researchers commented that turmeric was well-tolerated by all of the subjects.

In still another similar study, researchers at Baylor University Medical Center in Dallas, Texas, and Nirmala Medical Centre in Muvattupuzha, India, treated forty-five people with active cases of rheumatoid arthritis with curcumin supplements or diclofenac, a nonsteroidal anti-inflammatory prescription medication. Thirty-eight people completed the two-month trial. The researchers found that 1 gram of curcumin per day provided greater improvements in swelling and pain than 100 milligrams of diclofenac. Although there were no dropouts due to adverse effects in the curcumin group, 14 percent of the subjects in the diclofenac group withdrew because of side effects.

Cardiovascular Health

In Uttar Pradesh, India, researchers tested the ability of turmeric to lower lipid levels in 120 overweight subjects who were between the ages of fifteen and forty-five and had elevated cholesterol levels. For three months, one group of subjects took a turmeric extract and the other took a placebo twice each day before meals. By the end of the trial, the subjects taking turmeric had significant reductions in their lipid levels, including reductions in total cholesterol, triglycerides, and LDL, or "bad" cholesterol. The subjects in the placebo group had no significant changes in their lipid levels.

Animal experiments have also shown that turmeric effectively lowers cholesterol levels. Researchers at King Faisal University in Al-Ahsa, Saudi Arabia, divided twenty-four rats into four groups. The first group was fed a regular diet; the second group was fed a regular diet and black cumin seeds; the third group was fed a regular diet and turmeric; and the fourth group was fed a regular diet, black cumin seeds, and turmeric. The researchers found that the rats that were given either black cumin seeds or turmeric had significant reductions in total cholesterol and LDL levels. However, the rats that were given both black cumin seeds and turmeric experienced even greater reductions.

Gastrointestinal Polyps

Researchers at the University of Washington in Seattle noted that colorectal cancer has been associated with the consumption of a high-fat diet, especially a diet high in saturated fat. They decided to test the ability of the curcumin found in turmeric to reduce the incidence of intestinal

If you don't like the taste of turmeric or curry powder but want the health advantages offered by curcumin, the main ingredient in turmeric, consider using supplements instead of eating the spice. People report positive results from using either turmeric or curcumin supplements, but note that the amounts of these active ingredients can vary by supplement.

polyps in mice that were bred to develop polyps, growths that have the potential to become cancerous. Some mice were fed a high-fat diet and others were fed the standard rodent diet. The researchers found that when compared to the mice that were given the standard diet, the mice that were given the high-fat diet for three months had a 23 percent increase in the total number of polyps. However, supplementation with curcumin significantly reversed this accelerated polyp development. So researchers concluded that turmeric can help prevent intestinal polyps that may grow into colorectal cancer.

Neurological Health

Preliminary research at Michigan State University in East Lansing noted that Parkinson's disease is characterized by the clumping together of certain proteins. The researchers determined that a compound found in curcumin blocks the clumping of these proteins, which may have promising effects for people with the disease.

Certain medications used to treat the seizures associated with epilepsy may cause memory problems. Researchers at the All India Institute of Medical Sciences in New Delhi developed a study involving rats to learn if curcumin could reduce that side effect. The rats were divided into seven groups of six rats each and were given various medications for twenty-one days. The researchers found that curcumin reduced the memory problems associated with the epilepsy medications.

Two researchers in Egypt conducted another test on the ability of curcumin to protect memory in rats. For fifteen days, the researchers gave the rats one of four treatments: a high dose of curcumin, a lower dose of curcumin, memantine (a medication for Alzheimer's disease), or diclofenac (a common anti-inflammatory). At the end of that time, the rats were given a medication that causes memory dysfunction. The researchers then put the rats through a variety of tests to evaluate their memories. Interestingly, the researchers found that the lower dose of curcumin was more effective than the high dose of curcumin and the two other medications.

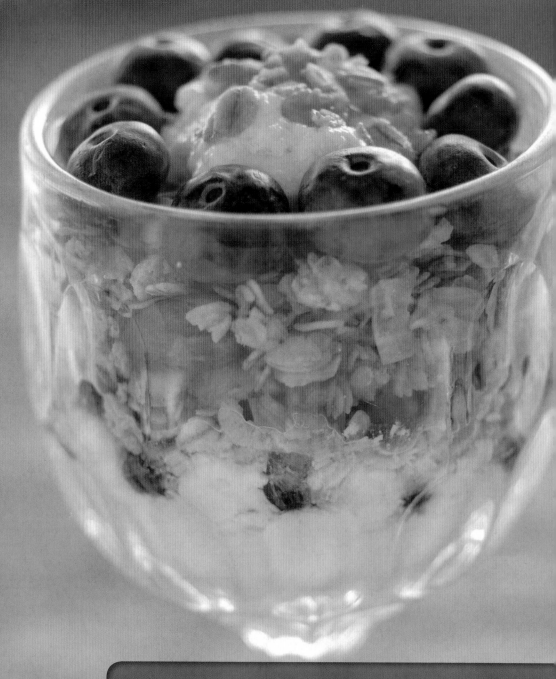

recipes

Blueberry and Yogurt *parfait*

This is an incredibly simple and delicious way to serve blueberries any time of the day. Try it for breakfast, lunch, a snack, or dessert.

12 ounces **vanilla nondairy yogurt**

1 teaspoon **agave nectar or honey**

2 cups (1 pint) **blueberries**

½ cup **granola**

Put the yogurt in a medium bowl and stir in the agave nectar until well combined. Spoon half of the yogurt into a serving dish. Top with 1 cup of the blueberries and ¼ cup of the granola. Repeat with the remaining ingredients in a second serving dish. Serve immediately or refrigerate until serving time.

47

beauteous Blueberry Salad

This easy-to-prepare side salad is a showstopper that earns rave reviews. The blueberries simply melt in your mouth.

2 cups **mesclun**

2 cups (1 pint) **blueberries**

⅓ cup coarsely chopped **walnuts**

2 tablespoons **extra-virgin olive oil**

1 tablespoon **aged balsamic vinegar**

Divide the mesclun equally among four salad plates. Top each serving with ½ cup of the blueberries and 1 heaping tablespoon of the walnuts.

Whisk the oil and vinegar in a small bowl until well combined. Drizzle 2¼ teaspoons of the dressing over each salad.

broccoli and Bell Pepper

It takes only a few minutes to prepare this nutrient-packed side dish, which makes it the perfect choice when you need to get dinner on the table in a hurry.

1 teaspoon **extra-virgin olive oil** or **avocado oil**

1 large **red bell pepper,** sliced

2 cups **broccoli florets**

½ cup coarsely chopped **walnuts**

2 tablespoons chopped **kalamata olives**

Heat the oil in a large skillet over medium-high heat. Add the bell pepper and cook, stirring occasionally, until soft, 3 to 5 minutes. Add the broccoli and cook, stirring occasionally, until tender-crisp, 5 to 7 minutes. Transfer to a serving dish and top with the walnuts and olives.

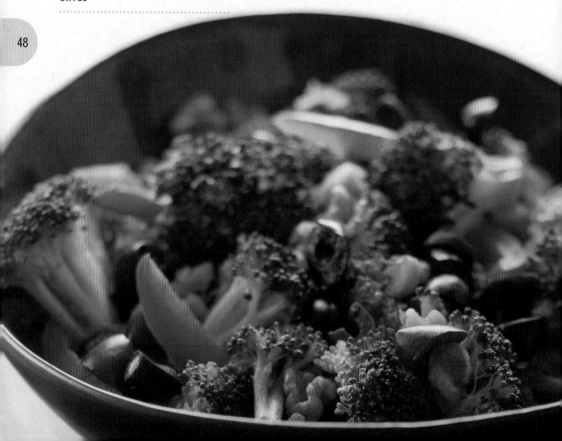

Broccoli Sprouts *salad*

This salad is as colorful as it is nutritious. Find broccoli sprouts in the refrigerated section of your market's produce department.

2 small **beets**

2 cups torn **leaf lettuce**

½ cup sliced **almonds**

½ cup **blueberries**

½ cup **broccoli sprouts**

¼ cup grated **vegan cheese**

1 tablespoon **extra-virgin olive oil**

1 tablespoon **aged balsamic vinegar**

Steam the beets until fork-tender, 30 to 35 minutes. Let cool slightly, and then peel off the skins using your fingers and cut the beets into bite-sized chunks.

Put the beets, lettuce, almonds, blueberries, broccoli sprouts, and cheese in a large bowl. Sprinkle with the oil and vinegar. Toss gently until evenly distributed.

49

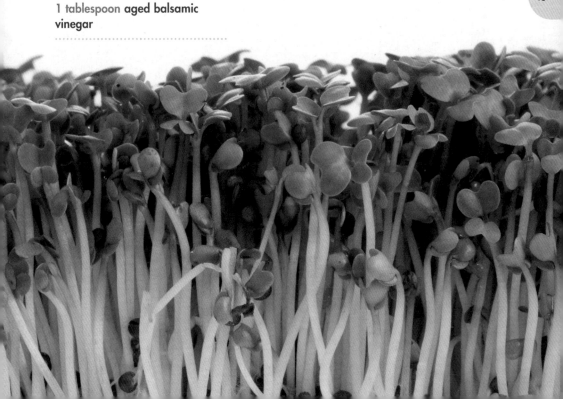

cranberry and Quinoa Sauté

Although cranberry dishes are popular in the fall when cranberry season peaks, this recipe includes dried cranberries, so it can be made any time of the year. The addition of quinoa packs this dish with protein.

1 cup **water**

⅔ cup **quinoa** (see note)

⅓ cup **pine nuts**

1 teaspoon **extra-virgin olive oil**

1 small **onion,** chopped

½ cup **dried cranberries**

Put the water and quinoa in a medium saucepan over high heat and bring to a boil. Decrease the heat to low, cover, and cook for 30 minutes. Remove from the heat, let stand covered for 5 minutes, and then fluff with a fork.

Preheat the oven to 325 degrees F. Spread the pine nuts in a single layer on a baking sheet. Bake for about 10 minutes, removing the baking sheet from the oven a few times to stir the pine nuts, until they're evenly toasted. Watch closely so they don't burn.

Put the oil in a large skillet over medium-high heat. Add the onion and cook, stirring occasionally, until soft, 3 to 5 minutes. Add the quinoa, cranberries, and pine nuts and cook, stirring occasionally, until heated through, 3 to 5 minutes.

NOTE: Because quinoa is coated with a naturally occurring soaplike resin that can cause bitterness, always rinse it before cooking (unless you're using a brand that has been pre-rinsed). Put the quinoa in a fine-mesh strainer and rinse under running water until the water runs clear and no sudsy foam remains.

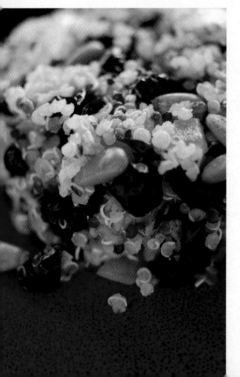

vegetarian tacos **with Flaxseeds**

Kids of all ages love these colorful and flavorful tacos, which are filled with one healthy food after another.

1 large **tomato, diced**

1 cup cooked or canned **black beans, drained**

1 large **red bell pepper, diced**

1 small **onion, diced**

½ cup sliced **black olives**

2 tablespoons ground **flaxseeds**

2 cloves **garlic, diced**

4 organic **corn taco shells**

1 ripe **avocado, quartered** (see note)

½ cup shredded **vegan cheddar cheese**

1 cup **salsa**

Put the tomato, beans, bell pepper, onion, olives, flaxseeds, and garlic in a large bowl. Stir gently until well combined.

To assemble the tacos, spoon one-quarter of the bean mixture into each taco shell. Top each taco with one piece of the avocado, 2 tablespoons of the cheese, and ¼ cup of the salsa.

Serve cold or warm. To warm the tacos, preheat the oven to 400 degrees F. Arrange the tacos carefully on a baking sheet and bake for 5 to 10 minutes, just until warm.

NOTE: To quarter the avocado, cut it in half lengthwise. Twist the halves apart and remove the pit. Cut each half in two and remove the skin.

51

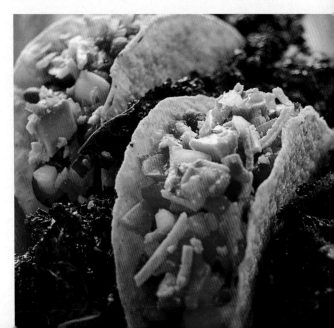

scrumptious Garlicky Peas

This is a dish for true garlic lovers. Though it can be made with regular or black garlic, make the effort to find black garlic, which is sweeter and softer than regular garlic.

2 teaspoons **extra-virgin olive oil**

15 **button mushrooms,** sliced

6 **scallions,** cut into one-inch pieces

10 cloves **black garlic or regular garlic,** chopped

1 package (10 ounces) **frozen peas**

Heat the oil in a large skillet over medium-high heat. Add the mushrooms and cook, stirring occasionally, until they release their juices, 5 to 10 minutes. Decrease the heat to medium, add the scallions, and cook, stirring occasionally, until the mushrooms are soft, 5 to 10 minutes. Stir in the garlic and peas and cook until the peas are heated through, about 5 minutes.

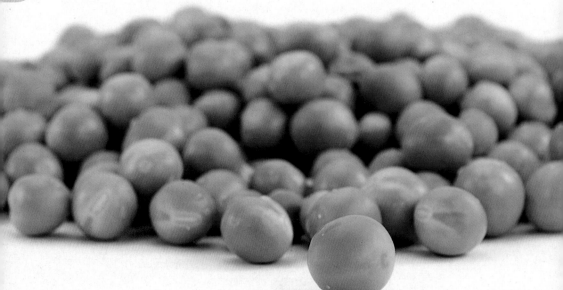

delightful Garlic and Vegetables

MAKES 4 SERVINGS

Garlic and olive oil are a classic pair, and there's no better time to use them than when zucchini, bell peppers, and basil are in season. This healthful mélange takes only fifteen minutes to prepare.

2 teaspoons **extra-virgin olive oil**

5 cloves **garlic**, chopped

2 **zucchini**, sliced

2 **red bell peppers**, sliced

1 tablespoon chopped **fresh basil**, or 1 teaspoon dried

Salt

Ground **pepper**

Heat the oil in a large skillet over medium-high heat for 30 seconds. Add the garlic and cook, stirring occasionally, until golden, about 5 minutes. Add the zucchini, bell peppers, and basil and cook, stirring occasionally, until the zucchini is tender, about 10 minutes. Season with salt and pepper to taste.

53

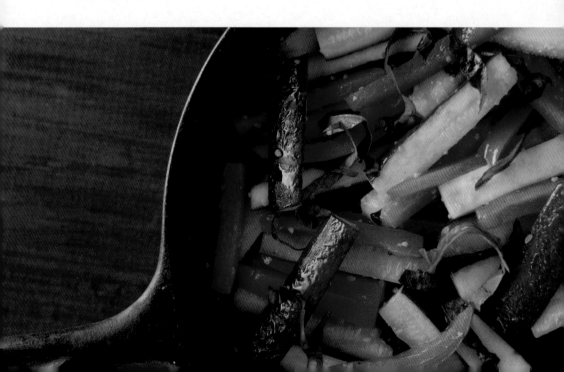

Kale *chips*

Store-bought kale chips are incredibly expensive, but there's no reason to pay high prices when it's so easy to make your own at home.

12 leaves organic **kale**

1 tablespoon chopped **garlic**

1 tablespoon **extra-virgin olive oil**

Preheat the oven to 350 degrees F. Line a baking sheet with aluminum foil.

Thoroughly wash and dry the kale. Remove the stems using your hands or a knife and tear the leaves into medium-sized pieces. Arrange the kale in a single layer on the prepared baking sheet.

Put the garlic in a small bowl. Stir in the oil until combined. Spread the oil mixture over the kale.

Bake for 8 to 10 minutes, until crisp. Watch the kale closely. If it starts to smoke, remove it from the oven, decrease the oven temperature to 325 degrees F, and continue baking until crisp.

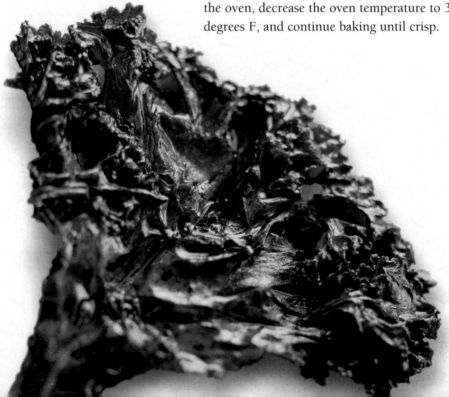

Super Simple *mushrooms*

Though it can be made with olive oil alone, this side dish tastes even better when it's made with both olive oil and red palm oil. Look for red palm oil online if you can't find it locally.

½ teaspoon **extra-virgin olive oil**

12 ounces small **button mushrooms**

2 tablespoons **red palm oil** or additional extra-virgin olive oil

1 tablespoon chopped **fresh thyme**, or 1 teaspoon dried

Heat the olive oil in a large skillet over medium-high heat for 30 seconds. Add the mushrooms and cook, stirring occasionally, until the mushrooms release their juices, 10 to 15 minutes. Add the red palm oil and thyme and cook, stirring occasionally, until the mushrooms are tender and fragrant, 10 to 15 minutes longer.

55

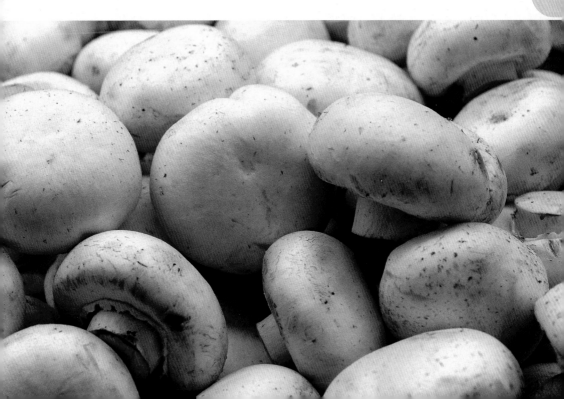

caramelized Onion and Tofu

Attention onion lovers: Here's a recipe that features not just one but two superfoods. What's more, it's super easy to make because the tofu is already cooked. Look for seasoned baked tofu in natural food stores or well-stocked supermarkets.

1 tablespoon **coconut oil**

1 large **red onion, or 2 medium red onions, thinly sliced**

2 tablespoons **agave nectar**

¼ cup crumbled seasoned **baked tofu**

Salt

Ground **pepper**

Put the oil in a large skillet over low heat until melted, about 2 minutes. Add the onion and cook, stirring occasionally, for 30 minutes. Stir in the agave nectar. Continue cooking, stirring occasionally, until the onion is very soft and caramelized, about 30 minutes longer. Sprinkle with the tofu. Season with salt and pepper to taste.

wakame and Chickpeas

This recipe provides an easy and inexpensive way to add sea vegetables to your diet. Plan accordingly: the wakame has to be soaked before using, and this dish must be chilled in the refrigerator before serving.

1 small bag (1.5 to 2 ounces) dried **wakame**

½ cup cooked or canned **chickpeas, drained**

2 tablespoons **toasted sesame oil**

Put the wakame in a medium bowl. Cover with water and let soak for 15 minutes. Drain in a colander. Transfer to a cutting board and thinly slice. Return to the bowl. Stir in the chickpeas and oil. Chill in the refrigerator for at least 1 hour before serving to allow the flavors to meld.

Turmeric-Spiced *asparagus*

Perfect when it's "just family" or when you're hosting special guests, this side dish features health-boosting turmeric. Make it with either fresh or frozen asparagus.

1 tablespoon **coconut oil**

1 tablespoon freshly squeezed **lemon juice**

12 ounces fresh or frozen **asparagus**

½ teaspoon ground **turmeric**

¼ cup sliced **almonds**

Put the oil and lemon juice in a medium skillet over low heat until the oil has melted, about 2 minutes. Increase the heat to medium and add the asparagus. Cook until just tender-crisp, 5 minutes for fresh asparagus or 10 minutes for frozen asparagus. Stir in the turmeric and cook, stirring frequently, for 2 to 3 minutes. Stir in the almonds and cook, stirring frequently, until heated through, about 1 minute.

57

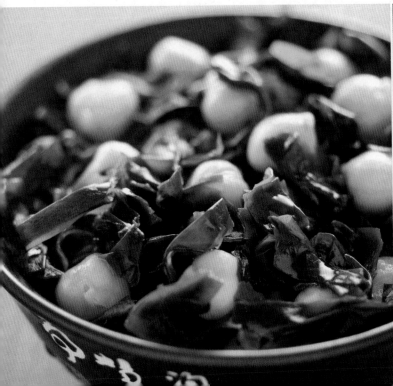
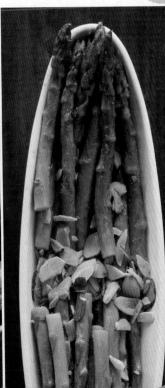

Yummy *edamame*

Young green soybeans are called "edamame" and are sold either fresh or frozen. To make this recipe, look for shelled edamame in the frozen foods section of your supermarket.

1 tablespoon **extra-virgin olive oil or avocado oil**

1 package (12 ounces) frozen **cauliflower**

1 package (12 ounces) frozen shelled **edamame**

½ cup shredded **vegan cheddar cheese**

Heat the oil in a large skillet over medium-high heat for 30 seconds. Add the cauliflower and edamame and cook, stirring frequently, until tender, about 10 minutes. Remove from the heat. Sprinkle with the cheese and let sit for 5 minutes, until the cheese has melted.

VARIATION: To cook this dish in the oven instead of on the stove top, preheat the oven to 400 degrees F. Put the cauliflower and edamame in an 8-inch square baking dish and stir to combine. Drizzle with the oil and sprinkle with the cheese. Bake for 15 to 20 minutes, until the vegetables are heated through and the cheese has melted.

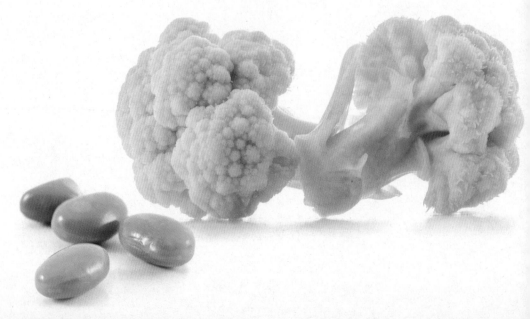

REFERENCES

Berries

Afshar, K., H. Stothers, H. Scott, and A. E. Mac-Neily. October 2012. "Cranberry Juice for the Prevention of Pediatric Urinary Tract Infection: A Randomized Controlled Trial." *The Journal of Urology* 188:1584–1587.

Krikorian, Robert, Marcelle D. Shidler, Tiffany A. Nash et al. 2010. "Blueberry Supplementation Improves Memory in Older Adults." *Journal of Agricultural and Food Chemistry* 58 (7): 3996–4000.

Moghe, S. S., S. Juma, V. Imrhan, and P. Vijayagopal. May 2012. "Effect of Blueberry Polyphenols on 3T3-F442A Predipocyte Differentiation." *Journal of Medicinal Food* 15 (5):448–452.

Neto, Catherine. 2007. "Cranberry and Its Phytochemicals: A Review of In Vitro Anticancer Studies." *The Journal of Nutrition* 137 (1): 186S–193S.

Broccoli and Broccoli Sprouts

Barnes, Peter J. September 15, 2008. "Defective Antioxidant Gene Regulation in COPD: A Case for Broccoli." *American Journal of Respiratory and Critical Care Medicine* 178 (6): 552–554.

Sharma, Chhavi, Lida Sadrieh, Anita Priyani et al. 2011. "Anticarcinogenic Effects of Sulforaphane in Association with Its Apoptosis-Inducing and Anti-Inflammatory Properties in Human Cervical Cancer Cells." *Cancer Epidemiology* 35:272–278.

Tang, Li, Gary R. Zirpoli, Khurshid Guru et al. July 2010. "Intake of Cruciferous Vegetables Modifies Bladder Cancer Survival." *Cancer Epidemiology, Biomarkers & Prevention* 19:1806–1811.

Yanaka, Akinori, Jed Fahey, Atsushi Fukumoto et al. April 2009. "Dietary Sulforaphane-Rich Broccoli Sprouts Reduce Colonization and Attenuate Gastritis in *Helicobacter pylori*-Infected Mice and Humans." *Cancer Prevention Research* 2 (4): 353–360.

Flaxseeds

Cockerell, K. M., A. S. Watkins, L. B. Reeves et al. October 2012. "Effects of Linseeds on the Symptoms of Irritable Bowel Syndrome: A Pilot Randomised Controlled Trial." *Journal of Human Nutrition and Dietetics* 25 (5): 435–443.

Demark-Wahnefried, W., T. J. Polascik, S. L. George et al. December 2008. "Flaxseed Supplementation (Not Dietary Fat Restriction) Reduces Prostate Cancer Proliferation Rates in Men Presurgery." *Cancer Epidemiology, Biomarkers & Prevention* 17 (12):3577–3587.

Pan, An, Danxia Yu, Wendy Demark-Wahnefried et al. August 2009. "Meta-Analysis of the Effects of Flaxseed Interventions on Blood Lipids." *The American Journal of Clinical Nutrition* 90 (2): 288–297.

Zhang, Wei, Xiaobing Wang, Yi Liu et al. June 2008. "Effects of Dietary Flaxseed Lignan Extract on Symptoms of Benign Prostatic Hyperplasia." *Journal of Medicinal Food* 11 (2): 207–214.

Garlic

Cope, Keary, Harold Seifried, Rebecca Seifried et al. 2009. "A Gas Chromatography-Mass Spectrometry Method for the Quantitation of N-Nitrosoproline and N-Acetyl-S-Allylcysteine in Human Urine: Application to a Study of the Effects of Garlic Consumption on Nitrosation." *Analytical Biochemistry* 394:243–248.

Ghalambor, Abdolazim, and Mohammad Hassan Pipelzadeh. January 2009. "Clinical Study of the Efficacy of Orally Administered Crushed Fresh Garlic in Controlling *Pseudomonas aeruginosa* Infection in Burn Patients with Varying Burn Degrees." *Jundishapur Journal of Microbiology* 2 (1):7–13.

Seo, Dae Yun, Sung Ryul Lee, Hyoung Kyu Kim et al. June 2012. "Independent Beneficial Effects of Aged Garlic Extract Intake with Regular

Exercise on Cardiovascular Risk in Postmeno-pausal Women." *Nutrition Research and Practice* 6 (3):226–231.

Williams, Frances M. K., Jane Skinner, Tim D. Spector et al. 2010. "Dietary Garlic and Hip Osteoarthritis: Evidence of a Protective Effect and Putative Mechanism of Action." *BMC Musculoskeletal Disorders* 11 (1):280–287.

Kale

Higdon, Jane V., Barbara Delage, David E. Williams, and Roderick H. Dashwood. 2007. "Cruciferous Vegetables and Human Cancer Risk: Epidemiologic Evidence and Mechanistic Basis." *Pharmacology Research* 55:224–236.

Richman, Erin L., Peter R. Carroll, and June M. Chan. July 2012. "Vegetable and Fruit Intake After Diagnosis and Risk of Prostate Cancer Progression." *International Journal of Cancer* 131 (1):201–210.

Tang, Li, Gary R. Zirpoli, Khurshid Guru et al. April 2008. "Consumption of Raw Cruciferous Vegetables Is Inversely Associated with Bladder Cancer Risk." *Cancer Epidemiology, Biomarkers & Prevention* 17 (4):938–944.

Zhang, Xianglan, Xiao-Ou Shu, Yong-Bing Xiang et al. July 2011. "Cruciferous Vegetable Consumption Is Associated with a Reduced Risk of Total and Cardiovascular Disease Mortality." *The American Journal of Clinical Nutrition* 94 (1):240–246.

Mushrooms

Cheskin, L. J., L. M. Davis, L. M. Lipsky et al. July 2008. "Lack of Energy Compensation Over Four Days When White Button Mushrooms Are Substituted for Beef." *Appetite* 51 (1):50–57.

Jeong, Sang Chul, Yong Tae Jeong, Byung Keun Yang et al. 2010. "White Button Mushroom (*Agaricus biporus*) Lowers Blood Glucose and Cholesterol Levels in Diabetic and Hyperchoˍlesterolemic Rats." *Nutrition Research* 30:49–56.

Mori, K., S. Inatomi, K. Ouchi et al. March 2009. "Improving Effects of the Mushroom Yamabushitake (*Hericium erinaceus*) on Mild Cognitive Impairment: A Double-Blind Placebo-

Controlled Clinical Trial." *Phytotherapy Research* 23 (3):367–372.

Signoretto, Caterina, Gloria Burlacchini, Anna Marchi et al. 2011. "Testing a Low Molecular Mass Fraction of a Mushroom (*Lentinus edodes*) Extract Formulated as an Oral Rinse in a Cohort of Volunteers." *Journal of Biomedicine and Biotechnology* doi: 10.1155/2011/857987.

Onions

Galeone, Carlotta, Claudio Pelucchi, Renato Talamini et al. October 2007. "Onion and Garlic Intake and the Odds of Benign Prostatic Hyperplasia." *Urology* 70 (4):672–676.

Jenwitheesuk, Kamonwan, Palakorn Surakunprapha, Kriangsak Jenwitheesuk et al. 2012. "Role of Silicone Derivative Plus Onion Extract Gel in Presternal Hypertrophic Scar Protection: A Prospective Randomized, Double-Blinded. Controlled Trial." *International Wound Journal* 9:397–402.

Kyle, Janet A. M., Linda Sharp, Julian Little et al. 2010. "Dietary Flavonoid and Colorectal Cancer: A Case-Control Study." *British Journal of Nutrition* 103:429–436.

Matheson, Eric, Arch G. Mainous III, and Mark A. Camemolla. July–August 2009. "The Association Between Onion Consumption and Bone Density in Perimenopausal and Postmenopausal Non-Hispanic White Women 50 Years and Older." *Menopause* 16 (4):756–759.

Sea Vegetables

Cooper, Russell, Charles Dragar, Kate Elliot et al. 2002. "GFS, a Preparation of Tasmanian *Undaria pinnatifida*, Is Associated with Healing and Inhibition of Reactivation of Herpes." *BMC Complementary & Alternative Medicine* 2:11.

Frestedt, Joy L., Michael A. Kuskowski, and John L. Zenk. 2009. "A Natural Seaweed Derived Mineral Supplement (Aquamin F) for Knee Osteoarthritis: A Randomized, Placebo Controlled Pilot Study." *Nutrition Journal* 8:1–8.

Jensen, Morten Georg, Mette Kristensen, and Arne Astrup. July 2012. "Effect of Alginate Supplementation on Weight Loss of Obese Subjects Completing a Twelve-Week Energy-Restricted Diet: A Randomized Controlled Trial." *The*

American Journal of Clinical Nutrition 96 (1): 5–13.

Shamsabadi, F. T., A. Khoddami, S. G. Fard et al. February 2013. "Comparison of Tamoxifen with Edible Seaweed (*Eucheuma cottonii* L.) Extract in Suppressing Breast Tumor." *Nutrition and Cancer* 65 (2):255–62.

Soybeans

Ma, D. F., L. Q. Qin, P. Y. Wang, and R. Katoh. 2008. "Soy Isoflavone Intake Inhibits Bone Resorption and Stimulates Bone Formation in Menopausal Women: Meta-Analysis of Randomized Controlled Trials." *European Journal of Clinical Nutrition* 62:155–161.

Rebholz, C. M., K. Reynolds, M. R. Wofford et al. January 2013. "Effect of Soybean Protein on Novel Cardiovascular Disease Risk Factors: A Randomized Controlled Trial." *European Journal of Clinical Nutrition* 67 (1):58–63.

Taku, K., M. K. Melby, F. Kronenberg et al. July 2012. "Extracted or Synthesized Soybean Isoflavones Reduce Menopausal Hot Flash Frequency and Severity: Systematic Review and Meta-Analysis of Randomized Controlled Trials." *Menopause* 19 (7):776–790.

Taku, Kyoko, Keizo Umegaki, Yoko Sato et al. April 2007. "Soy Isoflavones Lower Serum Total and LDL Cholesterol in Humans: A Meta-Analysis of Eleven Randomized Controlled Trials." *The American Journal of Clinical Nutrition* 85 (4):1148–1156.

Turmeric

Ali, Elham H. A., and Nadia M. S. Arafa. 2011. "Comparative Protective Action of Curcumin, Memantine, and Diclofenac Against Scopolamine-Induced Memory Dysfunction." *Fitoterapia* 82:601–608.

Madhu, K., K. Chanda, and M. J. Saji. April 2013. "Safety and Efficacy of *Curcuma longa* Extract in the Treatment of Painful Knee Osteoarthritis: A Randomized Placebo-Controlled Trial." *Inflammopharmacology* 21 (2):129–136.

Palve, Yogesh Panditrao, and P. L. Nayak. 2012. "Curcumin: A Wonder Anticancer Drug." *International Journal of Pharmacy and Biomedical Sciences* 3 (2):60–69.

Pashine, L., J. V. Singh, A. K. Vaish et al. April 2012. "Effect of Turmeric (*Curcuma longa*) on Overweight Hyperlipidemic Subjects: Double Blind Study." *Indian Journal of Community Health* 24 (2):113–117.

RESOURCES

Cape Cod Cranberry Growers' Association

cranberries.org

Cranberry Institute

cranberryinstitute.org

Highlights emerging facts about cranberries in the Cranberry Health Research Library.

Environmental Working Group

ewg.org

Publishes the *Annual Guide to Pesticides in Produce,* which features the "Dirty Dozen" and "Clean Fifteen."

Flax Council of Canada

flaxcouncil.ca

The George Mateljan Foundation

whfoods.com

Features information about the world's healthiest foods.

Mushroom Council

mushroominfo.com

National Onion Association

onions-usa.org

Soyfoods Council

thesoyfoodscouncil.com

Sprout People

sproutpeople.com

Sells seeds for sprouting broccoli and other vegetables and legumes.

US Highbush Blueberry Council

blueberry.org

Provides information on where to pick blueberries ("U-pick farms"), how to grow them, and endless ways to prepare them.

US National Library of Medicine

nlm.nih.gov/medlineplus

Allows users to search medical research by topic.

Wild Blueberry Association of North America

wildblueberries.com

Provides recipes, nutrition information, and details on how wild blueberries differ from cultivated blueberries.

ABOUT THE AUTHORS

For well over two decades, **Myrna Chandler Goldstein** has been a freelance writer specializing in health issues. She is the author or coauthor of hundreds of articles and ten books.

Mark Allan Goldstein, MD, is chief of adolescent and young adult medicine at Massachusetts General Hospital. He is also associate professor of medicine at Harvard Medical School.

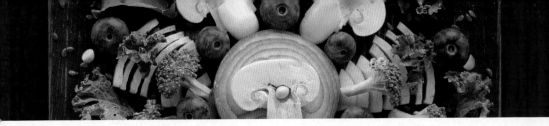

© 2014 Myrna Chandler Goldstein
and Mark Allan Goldstein

Food photography: Andrew Schmidt, 123 RF
Food styling: Ron Maxen
Book design, photo editing: John Wincek
Editing: Beth Geisler, Jo Stepaniak

ISBN: 978-1-55312-051-3

Printed in Hong Kong

Published by **Books Alive**
PO Box 99
Summertown, TN 38483
931-964-3571
888-260-8458
www.bookpubco.com

Library of Congress Cataloging-in-Publication Data

Goldstein, Myrna Chandler, 1948-
  Superfoods : nature's top ten / Myrna Chandler Goldstein, MA, Mark Allan Goldstein, MD.
    pages cm
  Includes bibliographical references.
  ISBN 978-1-55312-051-3 (pbk.) — ISBN 978-1-55312-095-7 (e-book)
 1. Natural foods—Health aspects.   2. Natural foods—Recipes.   3. Cooking (Natural foods)   I. Goldstein, Mark A. (Mark Allan), 1947-   II. Title.
  RM237.55.G65 2014
  613.2—dc23
                                                    2013035143

Note: Conversions in this book (from imperial to metric) are not exact. They have been rounded to the nearest measurement for convenience. Exact measurements are given in imperial. The recipes in this book are by no means to be taken as therapeutic. They simply promote the philosophy of both the authors and Books Alive in relation to whole foods, health, and nutrition, while incorporating the practical advice given by the authors in the first section of the book.

It is your constitutional right to educate yourself in health and medical knowledge, to seek helpful information, and to make use of it for your own benefit and for that of your family. You are the one responsible for your health. In order to make decisions in all health matters, you must educate yourself. With this book and the guidance of a naturopath or alternative medical doctor, you will learn what is needed to achieve optimal health.

Those individuals currently taking pharmaceutical prescription drugs will want to talk to their healthcare professionals about the negative effects that the drugs can have on herbal remedies and nutritional supplements, before combining them.

Self-Help Information

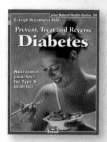

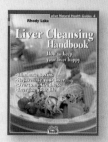

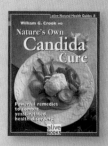

Healthy Recipes

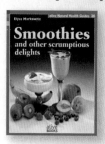

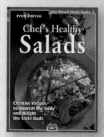

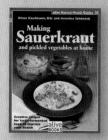

Healing Foods and Herbs

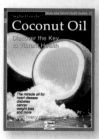

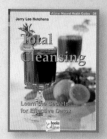

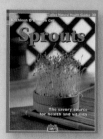

Lifestyles and Alternative Treatments

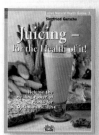

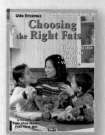

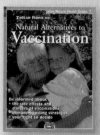

books
Alive

Summertown
TENNESSEE

1-800-695-2241 • www.healthy-eating.com